HOMEMADE HAND SANITIZER RECIPES 2020:

A Survival Manual to Protect Yourself Against Current Outbreaks and Counter Pandemics. Learn Smart Secrets to Keep Your Hands Clean and Healthy by Avoiding Germs

Grace Jessen

Homemade Hand Sanitizer Recipes 2020

Table of contents

CAPITOLO 1: INTRODUCTION 8
THE IMPORTANCE OF HAND SANITIZER 8
EFFECTIVENESS OF HAND SANITIZERS 11

CAPITOLO 2: WARNINGS AND CDC RECOMMENDATIONS 14
RISKS IN MAKING YOUR OWN HAND SANITIZER 14

CAPITOLO 3: HAND SANITIZER BASICS 18
WHAT'S A HAND SANITIZER? 18
REASONS FOR THE USAGE OF HAND SANITIZERS 22
WHAT CAN SANITIZERS PROTECT US FROM? 24
MISCONCEPTIONS ABOUT HAND SANITIZERS 26
BENEFITS OF USING HAND SANITIZERS 28
WORLD HEALTH ORGANIZATION SAFETY STANDARDS 31

CAPITOLO 4: IMPORTANCE OF HANDWASHING 32
WHAT IS HANDWASHING? 32
IMPORTANCE OF HANDWASHING 32
EFFECTS OF HANDWASHING 33
HANDWASHING VS. HAND SANITIZER: WHICH IS BETTER? 34
WHEN TO USE HAND SANITIZER. 35
HOW TO USE HAND SANITIZER. 36
PRECAUTIONS 36

CAPITOLO 5: EASY, NATURAL AND AFFORDABLE RECIPES 40
MOST GROUNDED HOMEMADE HAND SANITIZER RECIPE 40
FUNDAMENTAL OIL BASED HAND SANITIZER 41
WITCH HAZEL HAND SANITIZER 42
HAND SANITIZER WITH TEA TREE OIL 43
HAND SANITIZER WITH VITAMIN E OIL 44
HAND SANITIZER WITH DEMINERALIZED WATER 45
HAND SANITIZER WITH ROSALINA AND LEMON OIL 46

CAPITOLO 6: TYPES OF HAND SANITIZERS AND ACTIVE INGREDIENTS . 48

- ALCOHOL BASED SANITIZERS 48
- ALCOHOL FREE SANITIZERS 49
- RIGHT KIND OF SANITIZER 51
- ALCOHOL-BASED HAND SANITIZER SAFETY 54
- ACTIVE INGREDIENTS IN A HAND SANITIZER 55

CAPITOLO 7: DIY HAND SANITIZER GEL RECIPES 58

- CHAMOMILE OIL GEL RECIPE 58
- LEMON OIL GEL RECIPE 59
- SWEET ORANGE FLAVOR GEL RECIPE 60
- ALOE VERA HAND SANITIZER GEL 61
- ALCOHOLIC ANTIBACTERIAL GEL 62
- FRANKINCENSE OIL GEL HAND SANITIZER 63
- CINNAMON FLAVOR GEL RECIPE 64
- PEPPERMINT AROMA GEL 65
- BEAUTIFUL LAVENDER HAND SANITIZER GEL 66
- ROSEMARY AROMA GEL 67
- CLOVE ESSENTIAL OIL GEL RECIPE 68
- MOISTURIZING HAND SANITIZER WITH FRACTIONATED COCONUT OIL GEL 69
- NONALCOHOLIC ANTIBACTERIAL GEL 70
- SAGE OIL HAND SANITIZER GEL 71
- GEL HAND SANITIZERS 72
- ESSENTIAL OILS GEL 74
- GEL ALCOHOL-BASED HAND SANITIZERS 75
- STRONG NATURAL SANITIZER 77
- GENTLE HAND SANITIZER GEL 78
- TEA TREE HAND SANITIZER 79
- SANDALWOOD SANITIZER GEL 80
- VODKA HAND SANITIZER GEL 81
- LAVENDER VODKA HAND SANITIZER GEL 82
- TEA TREE & LAVENDER OIL SANITIZER GEL 83

CAPITOLO 8: DIY HAND SANITIZER SPRAY AND FOAM RECIPES 84

VARIATIONS AND SUGGESTIONS FOR CREATING DIY HAND SANITIZER SPRAY 84
EUCALYPTUS & TEA TREE OIL SANITIZER 85
TEA TREE OIL SANITIZER 86
NATURAL MOISTURIZING HAND SANITIZER 87
VETIVER OIL SANITIZER 88
CEDARWOOD OIL SANITIZER 89
CITRUS SANITIZER SPRAY 90
WHITE VINEGAR SANITIZER 91
APPLE CIDER VINEGAR SANITIZER 92
COCONUT OIL SANITIZER 93
OILS SANITIZER 94
NONALCOHOLIC HAND SANITIZER 95
LEMON-MINT ESSENTIAL OIL HAND WASH 96
WITCH HAZEL SANITIZER 97
CITRUS HAND SANITIZER 98
ALCOHOLIC ANTIBACTERIAL SANITIZER 99
LIME OIL SANITIZER 100
LEMON OIL SANITIZER 101
TEA TREE HAND SANITIZER SPRAY 102
LEMON OIL HAND SANITIZER SPRAY 103
VITAMIN E OIL SPRAY 104
PURE ALOE VERA SPRAY 105
USING PEPPERMINT ESSENTIAL OIL 106

CAPITOLO 9: DIY HAND SANITIZER DISINFECTANT WIPES FOR HANDS AND SURFACES 108

SWEET ORANGE NATURAL SANITIZING WIPES 109
NATURAL DISINFECTANT WIPES 111
ALCOHOL-FREE WIPES 112
VINEGAR BASED DISINFECTANT WIPES 113
GEL ALOE HAND WIPE 114
DIY NATURAL HAND WIPES 115
ALCOHOL-FREE HAND WIPES 116

TANGERINE OIL HAND WIPES 117
HOMEMADE ANTIBACTERIAL WIPES 118
DIY CLEANING WIPES RECIPE 119
DIY CLEANING WIPES RECIPE 2 121
DIY DISINFECTANT WIPES RECIPE 122
DIY ANTIBACTERIAL HAND WIPES RECIPE 123
IDEAS ON HOW TO CUSTOMIZE YOUR WIPES 124

CAPITOLO 10: ALCOHOL-FREE AND ALTERNATIVE HAND SANITIZER RECIPES 125

SAFE RECIPES FOR KIDS 125
ON GUARD OIL SANITIZER 125
ALCOHOL-FREE WITCH HAZEL SANITIZER 126
GERM DESTROYER OIL SANITIZER 127
VITAMIN E OIL SANITIZER 128
WHITE VINEGAR SANITIZER 129
APPLE CIDER VINEGAR SANITIZER 130
4 OILS SANITIZER 131
5 OILS SANITIZER 132
CASTILE SOAP & TEA TREE OIL SANITIZER 133

CAPITOLO 11: HOW TO BOOST YOUR IMMUNE SYSTEM 134

STEP #1—ACQUIRE A POSITIVE WAY OF THINKING 134
STEP #2—COPE WITH STRESS EFFECTIVELY 135
STEP #3—EAT MORE FRUITS AND VEGETABLES 136
STEP #4—DON'T DRINK ALCOHOL 136
STEP #5—EXERCISE DAILY 137
STEP #6—GET ENOUGH SLEEP 138
STEP #7—AVOID BAD FATS, EXCESS SUGAR AND EXCESS SALT 138
STEP #8—AVOID ILLICIT DRUGS 139
STEP #9—DON'T SMOKE OR DRINK TOO MUCH COFFEE 139
STEP #10—TAKE PROBIOTICS 139
STEP #11—ADD MORE PROTEIN IN YOUR DIET 140
STEP #12—MAINTAIN A HEALTHY SOCIAL LIFE 140

CAPITOLO 12: SECRETS TO PROTECT YOURSELF AGAINST CURRENT OUTBREAKS AND NEUTRALIZE PANDEMICS 142

How to prevent yourself from getting sick: 144
W.H.O Recommended Hand Sanitizer Recipe 149
Handwashing Technique 151
Indoor sanitation: the exchange of air 154

CAPITOLO 13: GOOD HYGIENE PRACTICES 156

CAPITOLO 14: CONCLUSION 170

Myths and Misconceptions about hand sanitizers. 177

Capitolo 1 : Introduction

Hand sanitizer refers to a gel or liquid with is used in decreasing infectious bacteria or germs on hands. They are usually available as forms, gels and liquids. Versions of hand sanitizers that are alcohol based usually contain a combination of ethanol and Isopropyl alcohol. And usually the most effective are those that contain at least 60 to 95% alcohol.

The importance of Hand Sanitizer

- You can use hand sanitizing liquid to clean your makeup brushes and ensure they are properly sanitized. Protecting the skin on your face from germs is just as important as protecting your hands, but other methods of cleaning your brushes might not remove all the bacteria. Simply saturate the bristles of your brushes with sanitizer and rub them gently in straight strokes for at least 20 seconds, then rinse thoroughly with water to remove all the makeup residue. Let your brushes air dry completely on a clean towel before using them again.

- Sanitizers will also remove most kinds of makeup stains from your clothes. Rub some sanitizer on the stain and then rinse with cool water. Be sure to do a spot test on delicate fabrics though, to ensure the sanitizer won't damage your clothing.

- Thanks to its alcohol content, hand sanitizer is very effective at removing those accidental pen marks from your skin. Next time you smudge ink on your hand, just use sanitizer as you usually would and watch those annoying ink marks disappear!

- Some of the ingredients in most sanitizers, aloe vera in particular, are great for soothing irritated skin. If you get an insect bite, swipe on some hand sanitizer to soothe the itch. It will also help reduce inflammation. Just be sure not to put it on skin that's been broken from scratching that will give you a nasty stinging sensation.

- Trying to get rid of that persistently sticky glue after removing a label? Rather than trying to scrape it off with your fingernails, just apply some sanitizer and rub it with a cloth. The sanitizer will loosen the glue and allow the residue to come off quite easily.

- One of the most germy, disgusting things we touch though we don't often think about it are our mobile phones. Between germs from your hands, face, and all the places you lay it down, your phone quickly becomes a virtual petri dish paradise for germs. Just saturate a paper towel with a pump of hand sanitizer and thoroughly wipe down your phone. Then you can get back to scrolling through social media more hygienically.

- Did you know that smell emanating from your sweaty armpits is actually caused by bacteria on your skin? If you find yourself in a smelly situation with no deodorant in sight, simply wipe down your pits with a bit of hand sanitizer so you can feel refreshed.

- More of us endure the annoyance of acne than we would probably like to admit. It always seems to pop up at the least convenient of times like when you're far from home and out of reach of your arsenal of facial products. If you find yourself in this frustrating situation, try dabbing a small amount of hand sanitizer on the offending blemish. Since acne is caused by bacteria, the antibacterial properties of your sanitizer will help to reduce it more quickly. Don't use this hack too often though, since the alcohol in sanitizer can dry out your skin if you overdo it.

- For those of us who are glasses wearers, one of the most annoying things that can happen is getting a smudge on our lenses. Chances are, if you're out and about, you might not have a wet lens wipe or a bottle of lens cleaner with you. But if you have hand sanitizer on hand, it works as a perfect substitute. Just apply a few drops to your glasses lens and wipe it gently with a soft cloth.

- Finally, hand sanitizer can also help you keep things clean around your home. From those pesky fingerprints on walls doors and stainless-steel appliances, to scuff marks and marker masterpieces on your walls for those who have children applying a bit of hand sanitizer and rubbing gently with a cloth will often do the trick. Just be sure to do a spot test first to avoid damaging painted surfaces.

Effectiveness of Hand Sanitizers

Just like washing your hands, the effectiveness of hand sanitizers depends highly on how you apply them. Sloppy and poor applications won't help you in any way except wasting your product, while a solid, thorough application will definitely help.

What's the definition of thorough? Health Professionals suggest to drop an abundant dose on our hands, not too think, not too dense, and then proceed to apply it over the entire surface of our hands, mainly between the fingers and spaces that look harder to reach, for a long enough time or as soon as the product is absorbed by our skin. Remember this fact, as it will maximize your levels of protection against viral agents and germs of all kinds, and it will prevent spreading them to other people.

Microbes cannot distinguish between commercial disinfectants and homemade disinfectants, according to the CDC. Disinfectants must contain at least 60% alcohol. If the handheld cleaner has an alcohol content of less than 60%, it will only reduce bacteria and not kill them.

Homemade Sanitizer recipes can certainly eliminate certain bacteria, but they will not work effectively if not well formulated.

Health experts warn that if done incorrectly, it can damage the skin rather than protect it from bacteria. Contents must use at least 60% alcohol to be effective, and it can also be used as a regulator against gravity. Although it is easy to obtain soap, it is more difficult to find many cleaning products such as disinfectants. Most experts agree that it is best to wash your hands with soap and water in the absence of Sanitizers.

Ideally, alcohol-based sanitizer helps to prevent germs by disrupting the membranes of different microorganisms, viruses, and bacteria, says James Scott, a professor at the Dalla Lana School of Public Health-- University of Toronto. According to him' some viruses do not have external membranes. What people may not be aware is that hand sanitizer may not be effective to many of viral infections out there. For instance, one study has even reported ineffectiveness against influenza B. In fact, the CDC explicitly recommends hand hygiene with soap and water as the first way to prevent infections before you use hand sanitizers for the average person. But the good thing is that coronavirus does have external membranes. And fortunately, it can be killed by alcohol as well as alcohol-based hand rubs," says James Scott, a professor at the Dalla Lana School of Public Health--University of Toronto.

So, hand sanitizers are a very effective option if you know you're on a busy commute and public transit and in another place where there are a lot of people and potentially a lot of germs. If there is no running water, hand sanitizer should have at least 60% of alcohol to reduce the number of germs.

Capitolo 2 : Warnings and CDC recommendations

Risks in making your own hand sanitizer

Is ethanol the best alcohol to use?

First and foremost, what is an ethanol? Well, an ethanol is also known as alcohol, grain alcohol, and ethyl alcohol, which is a vivid and colorless liquid. Due to the fact that it can eagerly dissolve in many organic compounds including water, it is also an ingredient in many products produced, beginning from paints and varnishes to fuel to personal care and beauty products.

It is also a common ingredient in various beauty products and cosmetics and it works as an astringent to assist neat skin, in lotions as a preservative and also to support to make sure that the ingredients in the lotion do not move in different directions.

As a result of the fact that it is effective in eliminating microorganisms like fungi, viruses, and bacteria, it is presently an ingredient that is common in various homemade sanitizers. In America, the Centres for Disease Control and Prevention (CDC) recommends people to make use of homemade sanitizers in places where both water and soap are unavailable.

It should be noted that it is highly flammable and one shouldn't make use of it close to open flames. Also, its inhalation can lead to you coughing or having headaches too, although it has been labelled by the FDA that is safe to use in any food product. Why is this so? This is due to the fact that it comes fully from alcohol.

Alcohol that is safe for the skin Products specifically for the skin are so sophisticated, with list of ingredients that are usually difficult to pronounce or very long. In terms of alcohol, it is usually perceived as unsafe for the skin, but it is also part of the ingredient that should be researched on Well, to cut the long story short, we are actually going to give in details whether alcohol is good for the skin or not.

With the fact that various individuals have imagined that every alcohol product are unsafe for the skin, well, this is far from the truth if you must know. There are various distinctive types of alcohols, with distinctive uses and distinctive health impacts. A few are considered to be safe when they are used, while some others are unsafe.

In addition to this, there are a few initial red flags to assist you know if your product, that is, homemade sanitizer, possesses a good or bad alcohol content. Assuming that you select a hand sanitizer and discover that the main ingredient is an alcohol, it is fair enough to say this is a bad product, and you might want to do thorough research before buying the product from your location.

Back to what we were discussing, it should be noted that fatty alcohols are derived from coconuts or nuts, which both of them are natural ingredients. These types of alcohols add cetyl alcohol which is originated from stearyl alcohol and coconut oil. Also, these alcohols are used mainly as emulsifiers; to assist get a luxurious and firm texture in hand sanitizers or any skin care product.

As a result of the high content the fatty acids possess, these types of alcohols have a good

Effect on your skin. It also possesses emollient properties, indicating they assist to increase your skin's defensive barrier by either safeguarding your skin from damage or locking in moisture.

Generally, fatty alcohols are considered safe, thus, when you buy any skin care product or any hand sanitizer and you see stearyl alcohol or acetyl alcohol, do not be scared.

Finally, it should be noted among individuals that when making use of any alcohol product, ensure that it is just a rinse-away product, such as cleansers. You should not use alcohols in products such as primers, serums, or even creams.

Alcohol that is unsafe for the skin the alcohols that are not safe for the skin are either denatured alcohols or simple alcohols, which are designed with the use of petroleum-based ingredients. In another meaning, it is something that one would not like to use on his or her skin or even bloodstream. These types of alcohols do not include isopropyl alcohol, ethanol, and alcohol dent. Many of them are often used as preservatives, while a few others are used as skin care formulas to the perfect textures, and also some are used to assist liquid formulas, and finally some of them are added in toners and cleaners to assist limit too much sebum.

Although, it might come with its benefit by having short-term impacts for people suffering from acne and also people with oily complexions, but they tend to dry your skin on the long run. When this type of alcohol is used regularly on a daily basis, it tends to weaken your skin's natural barrier by making the skin to be more difficult to retain elasticity and moisture.

It should be noted that these type of alcohol, when used regularly on a daily basis, can result to death, which can increase signs of aging like wrinkles and fine lines. These alcohols, when used on a regular basis, are also not likely to have an overall effect on your body.

Finally, these alcohols may have the ability of causing skin irritation, breakouts, and wrinkles, although they are highly unlikely to pose a more severe hazard.

Capitolo 3 : Hand Sanitizer Basics

What's a hand sanitizer?

According to medical and clinical professionals, our hands, whether covered with a glove, are the main way for the infection to spread or transfer the contamination of microbes. The use of hand disinfectants is part of the basic system for good infection management for people working in health center environments, or for those involved in aseptic processing in clean rooms.

There are many different brands and types of hand sanitizers, but some disinfectants have gaps in their effectiveness, and some do not meet the available European standard sanitization standard. Personnel working in hospitals and cleanrooms take many types of germs in their hands, and these microorganisms might be efficiently transferred from individual to personality or from person to gadget or surfaces that are significant.

Of those two classes, residential Flora is more challenging to eliminate. For critical surgeries, some security is given by wearing gloves. However, surgical gloves are not acceptable for all activities and, since they are not disinfected often or since they may be of defective design, they will end up contaminating on the move.

Additionally, It's not only required to use hand sanitizer before doing this kind of application, but it's also likewise essential that the cleaner effectively eliminates the large bacterial population. Studies indicate that subpopulations that are resistant to potential users can grow if a few germs stay after disinfecting.

There Are Lots of commercially Accessible disinfectants, together with the most frequent type being alcohol-based fluids or gels. As with other kinds of disinfectants, hand disinfectants are effective against different microorganisms based on how they function. In the most frequent alcohol-based disinfectants, the manner of activity contributes to bacterial cell passing through cytoplasmic discharge, protein denaturation, and ultimately cell lysis (alcohol is just one of those so-called "tissue destroyers").

A hand sanitizer has a comparatively low price, very low odor, and quick evaporation (restricted residual action causes shorter contact times). Alcohol also has an established cleaning effect.

When picking disinfecting hands, Pharmaceutical associations or hospitals should consider whether it ought to be applied to skin or lotions, or possibly both, and must be sporadic if needed. Disinfecting palms can be broken into two classes: alcohol-based and the more prevalent non-alcoholic.

Such factors affect both the safety and health of employees using hand sanitizers, since frequently alcohol-based cleansers may create excess skin dryness, and a few alcohol-based disinfectants can irritate the skin. Non-alcohol disinfectants are believed to prevent aggravation using hypoallergenic properties (with no odor and color) and components that provide protection and skincare via new petroleum.

Alcohol has been utilized as a disinfectant due to its antimicrobial properties attached to specific viruses and bacteria. To make a sanitizer working, it's imperative to combine water with alcohol to have a direct impact on germs, and the very best range is between 60 and 95 percent (most commercial palm disinfectants are approximately 70 percent).

The most commonly utilized alcohol-based disinfectants include chlorhexidine or hexachlorophene. Additives may also be inserted to hand disinfectants to enhance antimicrobial properties.

Hand Washing removes about 99 percent of temporary germs (although they aren't murdered). From then on, irrespective of whether gloves are not, routine hand Hygiene must be performed to remove all succeeding temporary plants to Decrease the probability of contamination from dwelling skin flora.

The hand disinfection technique is very important because its efficiency is not only related to alcohol, but it's also related to the rubbing technique. As an example:

Spread a little hand gel on your palm by pressing the pump to the pump. Put your hands together and continue rubbing the hand gel with both hands.

Pay particular attention to the following areas:

- Your fingernails
- The back of hands
- Both wrists
- In-between the webs of your fingers
- Your thumbs

Allow hands to dry. Usually, no more than 60 seconds are needed.

Routine use of hand disinfectants is needed before doing important activities. This is because alcohol is relatively volatile and does not offer permanent antimicrobial activity. Although it is easier to remove microorganisms from latex material than from the skin, regular frequency of disinfection of hands should still be used.

The safety of hand disinfectants is very low, and occupational exposure is relatively low, although it can accumulate indoors. Caution must be exercised when using disinfectants near open flames (which can occur when using a gas burner in a laboratory).

In short, personal hand sanitization is an important procedure that must be followed by everyone in their homes and offices. Hand hygienic sanitization is one of the main methods for preventing the spread of infections in hospitals and infecting them in pharmaceutical operations. This level of control requires the use of effective hand sanitizers.

Reasons for the usage of hand sanitizers

- Cleanliness

This shouldn't come as a lot of a marvel. One of the principal blessings of hand sanitizer is simply that: it sanitizes. Those products were designed to kill germs, and that they get the job executed. When used properly, hand sanitizers can kill 99.9% of the germs on your hands.

The Center for Prevention and Disease Control (CDC) recommends washing your fingers any time you're around meals (cooking it or consuming it), animals, garbage, and more. When you realize you are in these conditions, hand sanitizer is the best addition (or alternative) to wash your hands

- Portability

The last time someone tried that, they were disappointed. You can't just pick up a sink and take it with you. In those situations, where it's important to wash your hands, you won't always have soap and water available.

You may slip a small bottle of hand sanitizer in your glove compartment, a handbag, or even your pocket for situations where you would possibly want to wash your hands. Still, either can't discover a sink or awaiting one is inconvenient (think lengthy steps or away restrooms).

- Great for group settings

In the workplace, gyms, offices, classrooms, or any area with a great deal of foot traffic, germs spread fast. And even when you're not preparing to consume or carrying out the garbage, other people's germs may affect you (particularly in close quarters). That is why using hand sanitizer accessible is excellent for group configurations.

Teachers, students, and office employees can kill germs occasionally during the day without needing to leave their desk or classroom, and gym-goers may use a squirt of hand sanitizer before leaping on another workout equipment.

- Less risk for disease

Particularly during the Influenza season, If you take a little time to sanitize your hands a couple of times through the afternoon, you cut your chances of becoming sick.

Even a Fast trip to a buddy's home or the shop can introduce one to germs that might result in a cold, the flu, or Other disorders, so keeping your hands clean as possible is crucial.

- Softer-feeling hands

This could be among the most surprising advantages of hand sanitizers. However, it is not too good to be true. Hand sanitizers that don't include alcohol may actually enhance the feel of skin in your hands (notice that hand sanitizers with alcohol will not have this impact).

Some hand sanitizers contain emollients that soften skin, providing you with nicer-looking and smoother palms. You'll certainly see a difference in how comfy your skin looks and feels.

There are several advantages of hand sanitizer, from battling germs economically to battling them handily (and even enhancing skin). Certainly, employing this germ-fighting product frequently throughout the day will raise your cleanliness along with your health, regardless of where life takes you.

What can sanitizers protect us from?

Germs that cause things such as colds, strep throat, and other common ailments are responsible for the people seeking medical attention. These diseases also cause discontinuing work, college, and overall productive moments.

Many sanitizers are alcohol-based. It's made to be utilized when more conventional soap and water techniques of cleansing aren't available. When you put a small amount on your hands and operate the remedy in, voila, the bugs have been killed.

The alcohol at the hand wash triggers the walls of tissues to break down along with the virus or bacteria expires. It works in touch but doesn't provide you with continuing coverage. These regions contain surfaces like supermarket shelves, doorknobs, things at a shop that many others have touched, the cell telephone, and the list continue.

Sanitizers have lashes in them to help stop the alcohol from drying out the skin. It's as simple as putting on cream. This item comes in many different delivery methods. All are equally powerful. None need for towels or water.

You care about your environment and use soap washing, followed by regular hand washing with traditional hot soap and hot water. It is not suitable for palms that are soiled with visible dirt or other materials. If you're likely to be touching food items, you ought to use the gel and then wait for a whole 15 seconds for it to achieve maximum efficiency. You still will need to regularly clean your hands with warm soap and warm water into the very best germ coverage for you and your family.

Most of us don't wash our hands completely sufficient to prevent germ transmission. Water is not an alternative; both the FDA and CDC recommend a hand-held, called hand sanitizer having an alcohol content of at least 60 percent to work against the germ.

Harmful germ transmission, however, it's surely harsh on the skin. To fight the drying effect of alcohol, several have an additional aloe and vitamin E that assist in healing and soothing the skin. Another, not so renowned ingredient, is known as dimethicone.

It aids not only in curing, but also battling against skin irritation. Also, it can be present in ointments for diaper rash. Hand sanitizer, may be found in foam, spray, and gel foam forms. The gel takes a bit more time to wash than alcohol, and foam is not completely successful until it's permitted to stay on the skin for 15 minutes. Therefore, I favor gel to foam because of this.

There are a few additional Alcohol was used safely for several decades, so I would rather stay with the tried and true, as well as also the FDA and CDC recommendations everywhere. There are positive and negative germs, and we want both. Superior bacteria, known as "resistant flora," is useful bacteria found in the skin and in our intestinal tracts. Superior bacteria help stop bad bacteria from multiplying and causing us ill. Bad bacteria, known as "pathogens," trigger illness, parasites, and viruses.

The CDC recommends appropriate washing Of hands or a hand peppermint before eating, cooking, tethered to your baby, Helping the elderly or people with compromised health, administering health It is suggested that you wash or utilize hand antiseptic following using the restroom, diaper changing, taking out crap, picking up after a puppy, coughing and coughing, and managing raw food.

Misconceptions about hand sanitizers

Among the most popular fact is even though a hand sanitizer can ruin over 60 percent of flu viruses on your hand, many people actually contract flu from airborne representatives, by breathing at the germs. So, even if you are using a hand sanitizer, this could actually also be a powerful prevention mechanism for gastrointestinal disorders, rather than for disorders such as colds or flu.

Another myth is they are less successful as traditional handwashing with soap and water, also in removing germs from our palms. This isn't necessarily accurate.

Sanitizers lead to dry hands. These goods contain emollients, which are chemicals that reduce aggravation by protecting and soothing skin. You can make a marginally strong sanitizer in your homes.

But, if the product includes 60% alcohol, a generic producer could do the job just as well as a premium brand. It is not necessary to cover the higher price for a product with a new name.

The product includes 60 % alcohol; a generic manufacturer might do the job equally as great as a premium store brand. You do not have to cover the higher price for a new name product.

We may safely say that an alcohol-based sanitizer has become the best approaches easily to kill germs in our hands, but just provided that the item is used properly and responsibly.

An alcohol-based sanitizer is not only able to remove more germs than soap and water, but it is also gentler in your skin if used in moderate amounts.

Alcohol is not absorbed into the skin to a level to warrant these anxieties. Despite excessive usage, the level of alcohol intake is benign in the best. Alcohol can contribute to sanitizer dangers, but not to some huge extent.

The debate against alcohol content only holds up whenever the goods are used in a manner they weren't supposed to be used in. Employing example, an alcohol-based hand sanitizer is not supposed to be consumed. However, there have been several instances where kids, along with adults, have swallowed the liquid and dropped very sick.

Some producers have tried free of charge variations as a safer choice. Oils to neutralize germs, but thus far have not been as strong as alcohol-based hand sanitizers. If utilized properly, an alcohol-based hand sanitizer isn't any more dangerous in comparison to an alcohol-free version.

Benefits of Using Hand Sanitizers

There are a number of good reasons why using a hand sanitizer can be good for you. Here are a few:

- Hygiene

This should be like stating the obvious and not come as much of a shock. The mere fact that using a hand sanitizer simply sanitizes is one of the foremost benefits of using it. The ingenuity behind these products was to design them so that they neutralize germs; and going by popular opinions and research- based conclusions, they indeed do get the job done. It has been proven scientifically that about 99.9 per cent of germs are completely neutralized from the hands once the hand sanitizer is applied accordingly. The Center for Disease Control had advised the washing of your hands when you're around food, that is during or after its preparation; animals, public places, garbage, and so on. More than a few studies have established that the danger of spreading gastrointestinal and respiratory toxicities is reduced among families who use hand sanitizers. Once you find yourself in these situations or places, then a hand sanitizer is the seamless replacement for washing your hands with soap and water.

- Handiness

It is virtually impossible to carry a wash hand basin everywhere you go. So, in an event where you really need to wash your hands, water and soap might not always be readily available. It is far more convenient to carry a small bottle of hand sanitizer in the glove compartment of your car, your pocket or purse instead of having to deal with the inconveniences of either going about with dirty hands or having to join a long queue just to have access to soap and water. It's faultless for when you're grabbing a snack from an eatery after just coming out of a public space, like the stadium or Cinema.

- Good Option when Dealing With a Group

It is usually advised that you avoid being caught up in crowded places or getting too mixed up with too many people at these times. However, the reality remains true that you have to work, go to events, and be part of various groups. Germs about where foot traffic is heavy. Offices, lecture halls, public lavatories, you name them; they rapidly proliferate and spread. So, regardless of whether you are touching dirty stair rails or not, people around you can infect you with germs, especially when they are up close. This is why having hand sanitizer available cannot be overemphasized. So, people who are working together can neutralize germs every so often throughout the day without necessarily leaving their workspace or desk, and if you are at the gym, you can use a hand sanitizer before springing on the next workout machine.

- Lower Infection Tendencies

Decreasing your exposure to other surrounding germs either from people or places, is critical for your overall health, specifically during flu season or in times of viral epidemics. Do take the time to disinfect your hands every now and then throughout the day, this would help you drastically lessen any chance of you getting sick. A speedy trip to the salon or to pick up some groceries can expose you to germs that could cause various ailments; so keeping your hands as clean at all times.

- Softer-Feeling Hands

Surprisingly, this is one of the benefits of hand sanitizers. Studies have shown that hand sanitizers that are alcohol- free can really advance the texture of the skin on your hands. Hand sanitizers containing emollients will make your skin softer and give you nicer looking, slicker hands. You'll certainly see a change in how conditioned your skin would feel and look. Reduce the use of hand sanitizers that contain alcohol, as they may swab skin oils and cause skin cracking.

World Health Organization Safety Standards

Presently, alcohol-based hand rubs are the exclusively known means for quick and effective neutralization of a wide range of hypothetically harmful microorganisms on hands.

World Health Organization recommends alcohol-based hand rubs centered on the ensuing reasons:

- evidence- based, core gains of rapid- acting and extensive- spectrum microbial action with a negligible risk of engendering resistance to antimicrobial agents;
- Appropriateness for use in resource- restricted or inaccessible areas with an absence of the availability of sinks or other amenities for hand cleanliness;
- Ability to stimulate better- quality compliance with hand cleanliness by making the practice quicker and more suitable;
- Economic advantage by plummeting annual costs for hand cleanliness, representing about 1% of extra costs made by HCAI
- Minimization of hazards from antagonistic events due to amplified safety linked with better suitability and tolerance in comparison to other products

Capitolo 4 : Importance of Handwashing

What Is Handwashing?

Handwashing is simply the practice of keeping your hands clean from dirt, soil, and certain microbes with soaps and water. Handwashing is hand hygiene that can hinder the spread of water and airborne diseases like cholera and influenza. If you do not consistently wash your hands at appropriate times, you may risk contracting these diseases by touching the eyes, nose, and mouth.

Handwashing doesn't mean washing your hands at any opportunity you get. There are critical moments when you ought to wash your hands with soap and water - before and after using the restroom, before feeding a child or baby, before eating, before and after preparing a meal or touching raw meat, fish, and before changing nappies.

Importance of Handwashing

Handwashing is important health wise and otherwise. Every day, we are exposed to disease-causing organisms and infections that we can't possibly imagine. Washing your hands daily will keep you out from contracting these pathogens and prolong your lifespan.

Handwashing;

- Decreases the rate at which you contact respiratory infections.

- Minimizes the spread of airborne diseases.

- Reduce the rate of mortality in babies.

In medical practices, the importance of handwashing cannot be overemphasized. It's a hygiene practice that is totally necessary before the commencement of any medical procedure. Handwashing in hospitals will curtail the spread of disease by cleansing the hands of bacteria, viruses, chemicals, and microorganisms.

The prevalence of washing hands with soap and water is low in many countries of the world. For example, China has the lowest handwashing rate of 23% when compared to other developed countries. However, it is different in countries like Saudi Arabia and the United States, with 97% and 77% handwashing rate, respectively.

Effects of Handwashing

Handwashing is important, but frequently washing your hands with soap and water will lead to skin dryness. Also, it can lead to flaky skin conditions like hand dermatitis and eczema. It is also a symptom of Obsessive-Compulsive Disorder (OCD).

Substances Used In Handwashing

Water

Warm water is preferable to hot water and cold water and, as such, should be used in washing hands. When combined with a mild soap, it is more effective at removing soil, bacteria, and oils in hand.

Antibacterial soap

Antibacterial soaps have a list of antibacterial properties that are effective against microorganisms and bacterial in the hands.

Liquid soaps

CDC recommends that liquid soaps with hands-free control for dispensing content are more effective in removing bacterial and germs than solid soaps. Solid soaps may still hold up some bacterial and germs after use although, the transfer of bacterial is unlikely.

Ash

Ash is also a disinfecting agent like soaps. This is because it's alkaline. WHO recommends the use of ash as an alternative to soaps if the latter is unavailable. However, this is not to say that ash is more effective than soaps.

Handwashing Vs. Hand Sanitizer: Which Is Better?

The debate as to whether hand sanitizers should replace handwashing has gone viral and still is. However, it's worthy of note that there is a significant difference between the two in terms of effectiveness in killing germs, viral infections, and bacteria, and use.

Hand sanitizers, especially alcohol-based sanitizers, can reduce the number of microbes and pathogens roaming in the hands. However, not all types of germs and viruses can be reduced by hand sanitizers. Germs like cryptosporidium, clostridium difficile, and norovirus can only be removed by the use of soap and warm water.

Hand sanitizers work well in getting rid of many microbes, but it isn't effective when used in soiled and greasy hands. In circumstances like this, the use of soap and warm water is preferable. However, it is only after you have used soap and water that you use hand sanitizers.

The same thing goes for hands with harmful chemicals like pesticides. Hand sanitizers cannot remove this type of chemical. Instead, when used, the levels of pesticides on the hands are increased. In place of hand sanitizers, use soap and water to wash carefully before applying it.

The insistence of people using hand sanitizers in place of soap and water is totally wrong. In many cases, the two compliments each other. One precedes the other and, therefore, shouldn't be used to replace the other. Hand sanitizers only work effectively after you must have washed your hands with soap and warm water. However, if you are in a situation where there is the unavailability of soap and water, you can opt for the use of hand sanitizers with at least 60% alcohol concentrations.

When to Use Hand sanitizer.

Hand sanitizers should only be used when there is an absence of washing soaps and water. Also, if you want added safety after washing, you can use hand sanitizer.

However, you shouldn't use hand sanitizers when your hands are soiled greatly. When you have chemicals in your hand like pesticides, it's advisable you don't use hand sanitizers. Never should you replace the use of sanitizers with soap and water. Washing with soap and water is effective against viral infections, pathogens, and some dangerous chemicals that hand sanitizers have no chance against—for example, norovirus, closridium difficile, cryptosporidium, etc.

How to Use Hand Sanitizer.

Whether it's alcohol-based or not, foam or gel, it's not difficult to use hand sanitizer; a number of factors can affect its effectiveness.

• Ensure your hands are visibly dry.

• Apply the recommended amount in one palm and rub it together with the other.

• Rub in-between the fingers and make sure your entire hands are well covered.

• Once the skin is dry, stop rubbing the sanitizer.

This is the general use of hand sanitizer. However, depending on the product, there may be some variations in how such hand sanitizer should be used. It's essential to read the manufacturer's directions in this case.

Precautions

Alcohol is dangerous if ingested intentionally or not. Individuals seeking to abuse alcohol will likely ingest hand sanitizer. This could lead to death, poisoning, and the risk of fire. Alcohol is a highly flammable ingredient, producing a translucent blue flame. Some alcohol-based sanitizers may not produce this blue flame because of high concentrations of water and other moisturizing agents. Nevertheless, it's still flammable.

If a child is to use hand sanitizer, it should be used under the supervision of an adult. Other than that, it's necessary to keep it out of their reach. It shouldn't be rubbed around the eyes as it will cause inflammation. There should also be some restrictions placed on individuals (adults) who abuse or intend on abusing it to curtail access to these hand sanitizers.

The FDA raised the alarm about some antibacterial products causing some microbes to be resistant to antibiotics. This turns them into some deadly "Superbugs" in the names of MRSA (Methicillin-Resistant Staphylococcus Aureus) and Clostridium difficile. Triclosan, an active ingredient that is used in some sanitizers and washing soaps were reported to cause these superbugs. This led to the FDA banning the use of this substance in these products in 2019. Also, the European Union (EU) restricted the use of triclosan in various consumer products because of rising concerns regarding it. However, this does not pertain to alcohol-based hand sanitizers because triclosan is not a major ingredient that is found in them.

WHO and Centers for Disease Control and Prevention (CDC) in the U.S promotes the culture of using alcohol-based sanitizers often, especially in work and school settings. They recommend using sanitizers that have at least 60% alcohol content. Most products that flaunt the market reportedly have between 60% and 90% alcohol. However, that doesn't mean they are more or less effective.

The use of some alcohol-free hand sanitizers hasn't really been in line with WHO and CDC's health vision. This is because these products do not offer maximum protection against infections. Concerns regarding the safety of the chemicals used in these alcohol-free hand sanitizers have often led the WHO and CDC to discredit their uses. Like the triclosan, for example, if this antimicrobial compound is used, it may interfere with the proper functioning of the endocrine system.

The CDC recommends washing your hands with water and soap always, especially if have visibly your hands, after you have used the restroom and also before, during, and after food preparation. Wash your hands for at least 20 - 40 seconds with warm water and soap. For additional protection, CDC also recommends the use of hand sanitizer.

Hand sanitizers may not pose any threat to the skin, but they may strip the epidermis of oil, which will result in loss of skin lipid.

Capitolo 5 : Easy, Natural and Affordable Recipes

Most grounded Homemade Hand Sanitizer Recipe

The CDC suggests at any rate of 60% alcohol in hand sanitizer to adequately fight infections. This formula follows this rate and includes aloe vera for delicacy and basic oils for additional infection battling. This is the one I am right now utilizing after being in zones where infections are bound to be transmitted.

Ingredients:

- 2/3 cup scouring alcohol (70% or higher)
- 2 Tablespoons aloe vera (If you are unable to discover aloe vera, glycerin can be utilized as a substitute)
- 20 drops Germ Destroyer Essential Oil.

Directions:

1. Mix all ingredients and consolidate in a splash bottle (these are the ideal size) or little jug of any sort. Use varying.

2. Always check with a specialist or healthcare supplier before utilizing fundamental oils, particularly on youngsters or on the off chance that you have an ailment.

3. Using new aloe vera gel isn't as steady for counter stockpiling; a business brand is prescribed.

Fundamental Oil Based Hand Sanitizer

Fundamental oil-based hand sanitizer is a sort of sanitizer that doesn't utilize alcohol as one of its fixings. The motivation behind why certain individuals don't care to remember alcohol for their hand sanitizer is that it can dry the skin.

For basic oil-based hand sanitizer, you should gather the accompanying ingredients:

• 30 Drops of Tea Tree Oil

• 5 Drops of an Essential Oil of Your Choice

• 1 Cup of Aloe Vera

• 2 Teaspoons of Witch Hazel

• Washbasin

• Plastic Container (with a top)

• Spoon

• Cone-shaped tool or funnel

Witch Hazel Hand Sanitizer

1. Collect your needed ingredients.

A few people incline toward not utilizing alcohol in their hand sanitizer because alcohol emits a powerful smell and can have an extreme drying impact on skin. Utilizing a sanitizer containing witch hazel as its base is an incredible other option. Tea tree oil gives extra antiseptic advantages. Hence, this is what you'll require:

- 1 cup unadulterated aloe vera (ideally without added substances)
- 1 and 1/2 tsps of witch hazel
- Bowl
- 30 drops tea tree EO
- 5 drops fundamental oil, for example, peppermint or lavender
- Spoon
- Cone-shaped tool or funnel Plastic compartment

2. Mix the aloe vera gel, witch hazel and tea tree oil.

If the blend appears to be excessively faint, you can include a tablespoon of aloe vera so that the mixture will thicken. If it's excessively thick, include another tablespoon of witch hazel.

3. Mix in the EOs.

By now, the fragrance of the tea tree oil is powerful, so you can lessen this by adding other fundamental oils. Five or more drops ought to be sufficient, however if you need to include more, mix it in each drop in turn.

4. Channel the blend into the containing vessel.

Position the funnel over the opening of the holder and fill the container with the hand sanitizer. Top it off, screw up the lid on the top until you're prepared to utilize it.

• A little spray bottle functions admirably if you need to a handy sanitizer to bring with you daily.

• If you mix a lot for one container, spare the extra sanitizer in a container with a firmly fitted cover.

Hand Sanitizer With Tea tree oil

Ingredients

⅔ cup 99% Rubbing Alcohol

⅓ cup Aloe Vera Gel

5 drops tea tree oil

What you need

- A clean funnel
- Container
- Spoon

- Small pump bottle

Instructions

☐ Put ingredients in a container

☐ Mix all ingredients together

☐ Take the mixture with a spoon and pour it in the bottle

☐ Use a funnel if you need to

Hand Sanitizer with Vitamin E oil

Ingredients

6 tbsp 99% Rubbing Alcohol

2 tbsp Aloe Vera gel

1 tsp Glycerin

8 drops Vitamin E oil

5 drops Tea Tree oil

What you need

- A clean funnel
- Bowl
- Spoon
- Small pump bottle

Instructions

- ☐ Mix well all the ingredients in a bowl
- ☐ Store in a squeeze tube or spray bottle
- ☐ Use a funnel if you need to

Hand Sanitizer with demineralized water

Ingredients

6 tbsp 99% Rubbing Alcohol

2 tbsp Aloe Vera gel

1 tsp Glycerin

1 tsp Vitamin E oil

3 drops Tea Tree oil

Demineralized water

What you need

- A clean funnel
- Bowl
- Spoon
- Small pump bottle

Instructions

If you don't have demineralized water, you can let some tap water boil into a pot for a couple minutes, then turn off the heat and let it cool.

- ☐ Gently mix alcohol, aloe vera gel and oil in a bowl or jar
- ☐ Add demineralized water to achieve desired consistency
- ☐ Store in a squeeze tube or spray bottle
- ☐ Use a funnel if you need to

Hand Sanitizer with Rosalina and Lemon Oil

Ingredients

⅔ cup 99% Rubbing alcohol

⅔ cup Aloe vera gel

10 drops Rosalina essential oil

10 dropS Lemon essential oil

What you need

- A clean funnel
- Bowl
- Spoon
- Small pump bottle

Instructions

☐ Gently mix alcohol, aloe vera gel and oil in a bowl or jar

☐ Transfer to a squeeze tube or spray bottle

☐ Use a funnel if you need to

Capitolo 6 : Types of Hand Sanitizers and Active Ingredients

The hand sanitizers may be categorized as one of two forms depending on the active ingredient used:

• Alcohol-based

• Alcohol-free

Alcohol based sanitizers

This is a liquid widely used on hands to reduce infectious agents. Scrubbing your hands well is one of the easiest ways to avoid sharing germs and viruses, and to make sure you don't get sick yourself. But if you don't have access to soap and clean water, or if you're out and about and nowhere near a toilet, you're expected to bring hand sanitizer for health safety.

Another problem with hand sanitizers dependent on alcohol is the possible toxicity hazards upon ingestion. Many hand sanitizer dispensing mechanisms are very easy to open. They're also put to promote the use of open places. This is because the alcohol strips off moisture-retaining oils in your skin. The temporary absence of these oils on hands can contribute to increased skin irritation. It can also lead to

Dermatitis symptoms. Another concern is that alcohol in such items is toxic to floors and walls. The alcohol may stain the places where the dispenser can leak or spill.

Alcohol-based products have long been the recommended course of action by leading public health organizations such as the CDC, WHO, and FDA (second to hand washing). For hospitals and other health-care services, it is still the most used sanitizer. The effectiveness has been proved time and time again to withstand the test of time.. (Alcohol-Based Vs. Alcohol-Free Hand Sanitizers, 2020)

Alcohol rapidly denatures proteins at certain concentrations, essentially neutralizing all forms of micro-organisms. Generally, alcohol-free products are based on disinfectants, such as benzalkonium chloride (BAC), or antimicrobials, such as triclosan. The operation of the antimicrobials and disinfectants is both immediate and enduring.

Alcohol Free Sanitizers

Alcohol-free hand sanitizers can be successful instantly when on the skin, but the solutions themselves may become contaminated because alcohol is an in-solution preservative and the alcohol-free solution itself is susceptible to contamination without it..

The FDA removed Clarcon Antimicrobial Hand Sanitizer without alcohol from the US market, which found that the drug contained exceptionally high levels of contamination of various bacteria, including those that could "cause opportunistic skin and underlying tissue infections and could result in medical or surgical treatment and permanent damage." Gross contamination of any hand sanitizer by bacteria during fabrication would result in failure of the sanitizer's effectiveness and potential infection of the treatment site with the contaminating organisms.

Alcohol-free hand sanitizers came onto the market to fix gels issues and complaints. We have succeeded in many respects. Such methods are usually much smoother on the neck. In cases of accidental ingestion, they often pose much less of a threat. Hand-free alcohol sanitizers pose a low fire threat and are non-damaging to surfaces. Another obvious advantage of this is the increased defense that takes place. The ability of an alcohol-based drug to destroy bacteria stops after the substance has dried on the skin, but products based on benzalkonium tend to provide protection long after the solution has dried.

One potential downside with the alcohol-free solutions is that they come in the form of a foam most often. Although this typically leads to a more satisfying user experience, a special foaming mechanism is needed in the dispenser. This can make it prohibitive to upgrade from a non-foaming device, as new equipment will need to be mounted. Given some strong advantages in the health industry, alcohol-free goods have yet to gain significant traction. Alcohol-based gels tend to be preferred by health associations and are viewed by those in the industry as a more reliable alternative. It's not because the efficacy of benzalkonium-based approaches is not understood by these organizations. The word "alcohol-free" can refer to any number of on the market items. It's a vague word that makes the recognition of organizations such as the CDC and WHO unlikely.

Right kind of sanitizer

Both product forms do more or less the same job of destroying harmful microbes. By balancing your needs against your climate, budget and personal preference, you select the right product.

Effectiveness of hand sanitizers

Sanitation refers to a procedure using extreme physical and/or chemical methods to minimize numbers of microorganisms to a safe amount, without adverse effects on the nature of the product. However, many chemical sanitizers must be used for a sufficient time at high concentrations to achieve a desired sanitizing effect, which can carry some possible risks from chemical residues.

In addition, various bacterial states may exhibit various resistances to sanitizers, as in biofilms microorganisms are much more immune to antimicrobials than their planktonic state. Therefore, the selection of suitable sanitizers according to target bacterial states is important during food processing. More significantly, due to the stringent regulations, many chemical sanitizers are prohibited or restricted for certain particular food items such as organic food. (L).

In short, it should all be addressed when developing sanitizers for the food industry, bacterial organisms, bacterial states, and the related regulations. The effectiveness of the hand sanitizer depends on several factors, including how the drug is administered (e.g., quantity used, length of use, frequency of use), and whether the actual infectious agents present in the hands of the individual are sensitive to the active ingredient in the drug.

Interestingly, antibacterial soap is widely recognized as the worst thing you might use to destroy germs. It is because many but not all bacteria are killed by antibacterial agents, and then survive on the skin to allow the remaining bad bacteria to establish resistance.

Effectiveness

The efficacy of the hand sanitizer depends on several factors, including how the drug is administered (e.g., quantity used, exposure duration, frequency of use) and whether the actual infectious agents present in the hands of the individual are sensitive to the active ingredient in the drug. In general, hand sanitizers based on alcohol can effectively minimize populations of bacteria, fungi and certain enveloped viruses (e.g., influenza A viruses) if rubbed vigorously over finger and hand surfaces for a duration of 30 seconds, accompanied by full air-drying.

Specific effects have been reported for other non-alcoholic formulations, such as hand sanitizer SAB (surfactant, allantoin, and BAC). Nevertheless, most hand sanitizers are fairly ineffective against bacterial spores, non-enveloped viruses (e.g., norovirus), and unsystematic parasites (e.g., Giardia). Often, when hands are visibly soiled before application, they do not cleanse or sanitize the skin completely.

Enhanced exposure to alcohol-based hand sanitizer has been related to overall changes in hand hygiene in hospitals and health care clinics.

Safety Concerns

World Health Organization (WHO) and the Centers for Disease Control and Prevention (CDC) advocate the use of hand sanitizers dependent on alcohol over products free from alcohol. In addition, the use of alcohol-free products remained limited, partly due to the focus on alcohol-based products by WHO and CDC, but also due to fears about the safety of chemicals used in alcohol-free products.

Research has shown that certain antimicrobial compounds, for example triclosan, can interfere with endocrine system function. Another issue is environmental pollution from triclosan. Disinfectants and antimicrobials may also potentially lead to the development of antimicrobial resistance. In 2014, growing fears about triclosan led European Union (EU) authorities to ban the use of the chemicals in various consumer goods in the EU.

To be successful, hand sanitizers based on alcohol must have alcohol content of at least 60 percent. Some cheaper labels produce less and are no better than water. The worse scenario is that they provide false protection.

Sixty per cent pure alcohol, if swallowed, will pack a punch. Fortunately, as stated in the 2006 American Journal of Emergency Medicine, even emergency employees who use hand sanitizers do not inject discernible amounts of alcohol into their blood all day long.

There is a slight chance of a child being able to drink or lick a hand sanitizer based on the alcohol. This is something teachers and parents need to manage and monitor.

Alcohol-based hand sanitizer safety

Usage of alcohol-based hand sanitizers will increase as the cold and flu season approaches. But how effective are they and are they safe in preventing the spread of disease?

Hand washing with soap and water is an important way to reduce the bacteria in the skin and spread of infectious diseases. Washing, though, isn't always easy or practical, so hand sanitizers based on alcohol (ABHS) offer an alternative to soap and water. ABHS is available as gels or foams that primarily contain 60-70% ethanol, with a few isopropanol or n-propanol, or often a mixture. The germicidal mechanism of alcohol action includes denaturation of proteins and destruction of cell membranes, and all three have strong activity against bacteria, fungi and viruses such as common cold and influenza A viruses at concentrations between 60 and 80 per cent.

Given the widespread use of ABHS in infections such as common cold, there is minimal and somewhat contradictory proof of their efficacy in the population. One research found ABHS to minimize absenteeism in elementary school children due to respiratory and gastrointestinal illness, and compared to soap and water, ABHS was noted to cause less skin irritation and to be quicker, safer, and more convenient to use in another research.

For university students, frequent ABHS use decreased rates of upper respiratory tract disease by 20 percent and decreased days away from work or school by 43 percent, and daily use of ABHS also reduced coughing, nausea, and cold symptoms, as well as absenteeism of office workers due to bronchitis and diarrhea.

Active Ingredients in a Hand Sanitizer

Hand sanitizers, hand rub, or hand antiseptic agents contain 60 - 90% alcohol (ethanol, isopropanol, n-propanol) by volume. In addition, hand sanitizers contain;

1. Emollients and gelling agents that prevent skin dryness and irritation

Emollients are also called moisturizers. They are cosmetic preparations that are used for lubricating the skin, keeping it from being dry. They are contained in most hand sanitizers to prevent the evaporation of water from the skin by forming coats on the surface of the skin. Emollients can be used to treat skin diseases like dermatitis and psoriasis, which are products of frequent use of soap to wash hands.

There are different kinds of emollients - Petrolatum, castor oil, shea butter, stearic acid, cetyl alcohol, lanolin are some of the popular ones. Petrolatum or White Soft Paraffin (WSP) is known to be the most effective emollient.

Emollients may contain additional cosmetic compositions like fragrances, emulsifiers, antioxidants, humectants, etc.

2. Chlorhexidine

Chlorhexidine or chlorhexidine gluconate is an antiseptic that is used as a disinfectant. It is used for sterilizing surgical equipment before the surgical operation and disinfecting the skin. It comes in the form of liquid or powder and can also be used to treat mouth infections and prevent dental plague. Also, it can be used as an additive in antiperspirants, creams, and toothpaste.

According to WHO, chlorhexidine is categorized in a list of essential medicines as one of the safest and most effective medicines needed in the medical world. When mixed with alcohol (ethanol or isopropyl alcohol), it can prove effective against a wide range of microorganisms, fungi, and bacteria.

3. Quats NH4 derivatives.

Quaternary ammonium or quats are positively charged polyatomic ions belonging to the alkyl or aryl group. One of its derivatives quats ammonium salts and other quaternary compounds are used as surfactants and disinfectants and have shown to have antimicrobial activity.

4. Hydrogen peroxides for eliminating some bacterial spores.

Hydrogen peroxide is a chemical compound in its purest form that is used as an antiseptic, an oxidizer, and as a bleaching agent. It is an example of sporocides that is used for eliminating bacterial spores. It acts as a disinfectant and used for sterilizing surgical tools and is very effective against viruses as well.

Other compositions include;

5. A small concentration of water.

6. Fragrances and colorants.

7. Foaming agents.

Capitolo 7 : DIY Hand Sanitizer Gel Recipes

Chamomile Oil Gel Recipe

Preparation Time: 10 minutes

Materials Needed:

Bowl and spoon

Blender

Container for Gel

Ingredients:

2 cups of water

5 drops of Tea tree oil

15 drops of Chamomile essential oil

½ tablespoons of Aloe Vera gel

1 tablespoon of rubbing alcohol

Directions:

To produce Chamomile fragranced hand sanitizer, pour and mix all listed ingredients together in a bowl and stir well. Blend the mixture well and pure then into any container for future use.

Lemon Oil Gel Recipe

Preparation Time: 15 minutes

Materials Needed:

Bowl and spoon

Blender

Container for Gel

Ingredients:

2 cups of water

5 drops of Tea tree oil

5 drops of lemon essential oil

½ tablespoons of Aloe Vera gel

1 tablespoon of rubbing alcohol

Directions:

To produce Lemon fragranced hand sanitizer, pour and mix all listed ingredients together in a bowl and stir well. Blend the mixture well and pure then into any container for future use.

Sweet Orange Flavor Gel Recipe

Preparation Time: 15 minutes

Materials Needed:

Bowl and spoon

Blender

Container for Gel

Ingredients:

2 cups of water

5 drops of Tea tree oil

15 drops of Sweet Orange essential oil

½ tablespoons of Aloe Vera gel

1 tablespoon of rubbing alcohol

Directions:

To produce Sweet Orange fragranced hand sanitizer, pour and mix all listed ingredients together in a bowl and stir well. Blend the mixture well and pure then into any container for future use.

Aloe Vera Hand Sanitizer Gel

Preparation Time: 20 minutes

Materials Needed:

Glass Bottle

Container for Gel

Ingredients:

Tea tree essential oil – 20 drops

Lavender essential oil – 20 dr0ps

Rubbing alcohol – ¼

Aloe vera gel

Directions:

Fill your glass bottle with ¼ rubbing alcohol

Add the essential oils

Then fill the rest of the bottle with the aloe vera gel.

Shake well before you use it.

Alcoholic Antibacterial Gel

Preparation Time: 15 minutes

Materials Needed:

Bottle

Container for Gel / Jar

Ingredients:

1/3 aloe vera gel

2/3 bottle ethanol

5 drops peppermint essential oil

10 drops lemon essential oil

Directions:

If you do not have the gel purchased, cut an aloe vera leaf from a plant you have and prepare it. Pour the aloe vera gel into the container until it is ⅓ full.

Add the alcohol, close the bottle, and stir well so that the two ingredients are integrated.

Open the container again and add the drops of essential oils.

Mix everything well so that there is a homogeneous gel.

Store it in a jar or bottle with a dispenser or small opening for easy use when you need it, and the natural antibacterial gel is ready to go!

Frankincense Oil Gel Hand Sanitizer

Preparation Time: 20 minutes

Materials Needed:

Bowl and spoon

Container for Gel

Ingredients:

Rubbing alcohol - 1 tablespoon

Aloe vera gel - ½ tablespoons

Frankincense essential oil - 10 drops

Tea tree oil - 5 drops

Water (filtered) 2 cups

Directions:

Mix all the ingredients in a cup or bowl, then pour them into a bottle for everyday use.

Cinnamon Flavor Gel Recipe

Preparation Time: 20 minutes

Materials Needed:

Bowl and spoon

Container for Gel

Ingredients:

Rubbing alcohol - 1 tablespoon

Aloe vera gel - ½ tablespoons

Cinnamon essential oil .- 5 drops

Tea tree oil . 5 drops

Water (filtered) 2 cups

Directions:

We need to mix all of the ingredients together to create our hygienic gel and use it for every occasion.

Peppermint Aroma Gel

Preparation Time: 20 minutes

Materials Needed:

Bowl and spoon

Container for Gel

Ingredients:

Rubbing alcohol - 1 tablespoon

Aloe vera gel - ½ tablespoons

Peppermint essential oil - 15 drops

Tea tree oil - 5 drops

Water (filtered) 2 cups

Directions:

We need to mix all of the ingredients together to create our hygienic gel and use it for every occasion.

Beautiful Lavender Hand Sanitizer Gel

Preparation Time: 20 minutes

Materials Needed:

Bowl and spoon

Container for Gel

Ingredients:

Rubbing alcohol - 2 tablespoons

Aloe vera gel - ½ tablespoons

Lavender essential oil - 20 drops

Tea tree oil - 5 drops

Water filtered - 2 cups

Directions:

We need to mix all of the ingredients together to create our hygienic gel and use it for every occasion.

Rosemary Aroma Gel

Preparation Time: 20 minutes

Materials Needed:

Bowl and spoon

Container for Gel

Ingredients:

Rubbing alcohol - 2 tablespoons

Aloe vera gel - ½ tablespoons

Rosemary essential oil . 15 drops

Tea tree oil - 5 drops

Water (filtered) - 2 cups

Directions:

We need to mix all of the ingredients together to create our hygienic gel and use it for every occasion.

Clove Essential Oil Gel Recipe

Preparation Time: 20 minutes

Materials Needed:

Bowl and spoon

Container for Gel

Ingredients:

Rubbing alcohol - 2 tablespoons

Aloe vera gel - ½ tablespoons

Clove essential oil .- 20 drops

Tea tree oil - 5 drops

Water (filtered) - 2 cups

Directions:

We need to mix all of the ingredients together to create our hygienic gel and use it for every occasion.

Moisturizing Hand Sanitizer with Fractionated Coconut Oil Gel

Preparation Time: 20 minutes

Materials Needed:

Bowl and spoon

Container for Gel

Ingredients:

2/3 cup (158 ml. / 5.3 fl. oz) isopropyl alcohol (99% rubbing alcohol)

1/3 cup (79 ml. / 2.7 fl. oz) aloe vera gel

1 tsp. (5 ml) fractionated coconut oil

Directions:

In a small mason jar or container, mix the alcohol and aloe vera gel together. Then mix in the fractionated coconut oil. Put the lid on the jar and shake vigorously to ensure it mixes well. Then pour into a container of your choice.

**Note: Solid coconut oil, like that commonly used for cooking, will NOT work here. Fractionated coconut oil has been distilled and had fatty acids removed, which allows it to stay in liquid form. It's more easily absorbed by your skin, and importantly, has a long shelf life!

Nonalcoholic Antibacterial Gel

Preparation Time: 20 minutes

Materials Needed:

Bowl and spoon

Container for Gel

Ingredients:: 30 ml rosemary water

1/2 tbsp vegetable glycerin - 5 drops eucalyptus essential oil

5 drops lavender essential oil - 5 drops lemon essential oil

Directions:

Prepare the glycerin according to the directions on the package.

If you do not buy it, prepare the rosemary water by making an infusion in quantity so that you have at the end the 30 ml of rosemary water well concentrated.

In the bottle in which you are going to store this natural antibacterial gel put the glycerin (you can make several jars if you want to have it in small pots to carry on top).

Add the rosemary water and mix with a stick or wooden kitchen spoon.

Add the essential oils and mix again until you see that there is a homogeneous gel.

Transfer to an empty and clean bottle for use.

Sage Oil Hand Sanitizer Gel

Preparation Time: 20 minutes

Materials Needed:

Bowl and spoon

Container for Gel

Ingredients:

Sage essential oil – 10 drops

Isopropyl alcohol (not less than 70%) – 1 cup

Aloe vera gel – ½ cup

Tea tree oil – 15 drops

Directions:

Mix all your ingredients in a bowl, then transfer to a tube or container.

Gel Hand Sanitizers

Preparation Time: 15 minutes

Materials Needed:

Bowl and spoon

Container for Gel

Ingredients:

Ingredients for the third recipe are given below:

One cup of alcohol (91% Isopropyl)

Half cup of the aloe vera gel (Natural)

Fifteen drops of the tea tree oil (You can use any other essential oil that is antibacterial)

Directions:

Using the pouring spout, pour the alcohol into a container. Some people are using vodka as well instead of alcohol, but that is not effective when compared with alcohol. The percentage of alcohol in vodka is very less.

Pour the aloe vera gel in the mixture, but make sure that you carefully measure the gel before mixing it into the batter. If you are using alcohol alone, it can be hard for your hands; however, the addition of the aloe vera gel makes the mixture smooth. Make sure that the gel used in the sanitizer is natural, and you can use the gel straight from the plant. The alcohol in the mixture will now act as a preservative. However, keep it in your mind that using the natural aloe vera gel will make the final product thicker. When you are using this sanitizer, you need to rub your hands carefully.

Now add the essential oil in it. We are using the tea tree oil because of its antibacterial properties. You can use some other essential oils as well if you don't like the smell of the tea tree oil. Some other essential oils which can be used are lemongrass, lavender, or eucalyptus.

Stirring won't be enough in this case due to the thickness of the gel. You need to whisk the whole mixture. Beat the hand sanitizer into it to create a gel.

Now, the final step is to sanitize the bottles in which you want to keep this gel and then pour in the sanitizer.

Don't forget to label the sanitizer; anyone from your home can ingest the hand sanitizer, so care is critical. After marking it, you are ready to use it.

Precautions

Make sure that you are using natural ingredients for this gel; avoid using the aloe vera gel available in the market. You need thick gel for this hand sanitizer if you want good results from it.

Essential Oils Gel

Preparation Time: 20 minutes

Materials Needed:

Bowl and spoon

Container for Gel

Ingredients:

Aloe vera gel ¼ cup

Orange essential oil - 20 drops

Clove essential oil - 5 drops

Cinnamon Essential oil - 10 drops

Lavender essential oil - 10 drops

Rosemary essential oil. - 5 drops

Directions:

Mix all the ingredients in a cup or bowl, then pour them into a bottle for everyday use.

Gel Alcohol-based Hand Sanitizers

Preparation Time: 20 minutes

Materials Needed:

Bowl and spoon

Container for Gel

Ingredients:

⅓ cup of aloe vera gel.

⅔ cup of Isopropyl or rubbing alcohol with 91% purity at the minimum.

Spoon.

Mixing bowl.

Funnel.

Container or bottle

Directions:

Add aloe vera gel and isopropyl alcohol into a mixing bowl.

Use spoon to stir until it's evenly mixed.

Pour the mixture over a funnel into the container or bottle and replace the lid.

Shake before use.

If you plan on adding essential oils into your hand sanitizers, you need to understand what each essential oil does. You can choose to combine two or more oils or decide to just use one. By adding them, you will have an amazing aromatic experience, while also keeping yourself safe from germs.

What you need to know about essential oils

Lavender oil smells nice and is known to have antibacterial and antiviral properties. It helps to reduce migraines and minor irritations around the skin.

Lemongrass oil is known to have antibacterial and antifungal properties.

Tea tree oil is known to have antifungal, antiseptic, antiviral, and antibacterial properties.

Cinnamon oil has a fragrance that will enhance your concentration and reduce drowsiness. It can also reduce headaches.

Rosemary essential is known to boost alertness and memory.

Peppermint essential oil has a compelling scent that soothes the nerves and enhances mental clarity.

Vitamin E keeps the skin fresh and act as a moisturizer, just like aloe vera gel.

Strong Natural Sanitizer

Preparation Time: 20 minutes

Materials Needed:

Bowl and spoon

Container for Gel

Ingredients

⅔ Cup rubbing alcohol 70 percent or higher

2 tablespoons Aloe Vera (Glycerin may be used as a substitute)

20 Drops of germ destroyer essential oil (Germ fighter essential oil is stronger but may not be safe for use with kids)

Directions:

First add the Aloe Vera or Glycerin to the kitchen bowl. Afterwards measure out the rubbing alcohol in a ⅔ measuring up and use it to rinse the tablespoon the aloe vera gel or glycerin was in. After rinsing the tablespoon into the bowl with the rubbing alcohol stir the mixture with a spoon. Add the germ destroyer essential oil to the mix next. Stir the mixture again. Package the mixture into the desired container.

Gentle Hand Sanitizer Gel

Preparation Time: 15 minutes

Materials Needed:

Bowl and spoon

Container for Gel

Ingredients:

A Bowl and a Spoon

A Funnel

Reusable Silicon Tube

Also prepare the following materials:

¼ cup aloe vera gel

20 drops germ destroyer essential oil

Directions:

Mix all the ingredients in the bowl, using the spoon. Once it's all mixed nicely, use the funnel to pour it into reusable silicon tube.

Tea Tree Hand Sanitizer

Preparation Time: 15 minutes

Materials Needed:

Bowl and spoon

Container for Gel

Ingredients:

2 tablespoons of coconut oil

10 tablespoons of sunflower oil

5 tablespoons of potassium chloride

10-20 drops of Tea Trea Oil for sanitizing

2 cups of Strong Acidic Water 2.5pH for sanitizing (prefered) or 2 cups of purified boiled water

Directions:

Pour the sunflower and coconut oil into a pot and put on high heat.

Mix potassium chloride with purified water in a separate pot and then add to the pot with oils.

Mix together using a hand-held stick blender on low until you create a paste. Pour the purified water into the pot and combine using the stick blender.

Sandalwood Sanitizer Gel

Preparation Time: 10 minutes

Materials Needed:

Bowl and spoon

Container for Gel

Ingredients:

5 drops sandalwood essential oil

5 drops tea tree oil

1 tablespoon rubbing alcohol

½ tablespoons aloe vera gel

2 cups boiled and cooled water

Directions:

In a glass bowl, add the essential oil, tree oil and rubbing alcohol and stir to combine.

Add the aloe vera gel and mix until well combined.

Now, add the water and mix until well combined.

Through a funnel, pour the hand sanitizer into small, clean squirt bottles.

Store in a cool place out of direct sunlight.

Remember to shake gently before each use.

Vodka Hand Sanitizer Gel

Preparation Time: 15 minutes

Materials Needed:

Bowl and spoon

Container for Gel

Ingredients:

4 tbsp. (60 ml. / 2 fl. oz.) 180-proof vodka (or higher)

1 tsp. (5 ml.) aloe vera gel

1/2 tsp. (2.5 ml.) vitamin E oil

optional: 10-12 drops essential oils of your choice

Directions:

Put the vodka, aloe vera gel, and vitamin E oil in a small bowl or jar and mix well. If using an essential oil, add a few drops at a time, stirring slowly. Store in an airtight container of your choice.

Lavender Vodka Hand Sanitizer Gel

Preparation Time: 15 minutes

Materials Needed:

Bowl and spoon

Container for Gel

Ingredients:

4 tbsp. (60 ml. / 2 fl. oz.) 180-proof vodka (or higher)

15 drops of vegetable glycerin

6 drops of lavender essential oil

Directions:

Put the vodka and vegetable glycerin in a small jar or container and mix well. Slowly add the lavender essential oil as you stir gently. Store in a container of your choice.

Note: It is VERY important to check the proof of your vodka. If it it's not at least 180-proof, the alcohol content won't be sufficient to kill germs.

Tea Tree & Lavender Oil Sanitizer Gel

Preparation Time: 10 minutes

Materials Needed:

Bowl and spoon

Container for Gel

Ingredients:

20 drops lavender essential oil

5 drops tea tree oil

2 tablespoons rubbing alcohol

½ tablespoons aloe vera gel

2 cups boiled and cooled water

Directions:

In a glass bowl, add the essential oil, tree oil and rubbing alcohol and stir to combine.

Add the aloe vera gel and mix until well combined.

Now, add the water and mix until well combined.

Through a funnel, pour the hand sanitizer into small, clean squirt bottles.

Store in a cool place out of direct sunlight.

Remember to shake gently before each use.

Capitolo 8 : DIY Hand Sanitizer Spray and Foam Recipes

Variations and Suggestions for Creating DIY Hand Sanitizer Spray

You are able to include 1/4 tsp of Vitamin E Oil for a hand sanitizer spray in order to add moisture back in your palms with every use.

If you want to generate a natural hand sanitizer spray, then you may use Witch Hazel instead of this alcohol. Witch Hazel is alcohol-free and can provide you a far milder hand sanitizer with no strong alcohol odor. If you would like a powerful sanitizer that resembles the store-bought, I suggest sticking with the rubbing alcohol variant over, rather than the milder version.

The aloe vera in this recipe must help stop your hands from drying out up to the hand sanitizers. If you discover the hand sanitizer is beginning to dry out of your hands, you might choose to take a little container of Homemade Lotion to utilize after implementing the sanitizer. This can help restore the warmth on your hands and give them a more agreeable smell!

Eucalyptus & Tea Tree Oil Sanitizer

Preparation Time: 10 minute

Materials Needed:

Bowl and Spoon

Funnel

Squirt Bottles

Ingredients:: 15 drops eucalyptus essential oil

5 drops tea tree oil

1 tablespoon rubbing alcohol

½ tablespoons aloe vera gel

2 cups boiled and cooled water

Directions:

In a glass bowl, add the essential oil, tree oil and rubbing alcohol and stir to combine.

Add the aloe vera gel and mix until well combined.

Now, add the water and mix until well combined.

Through a funnel, pour the hand sanitizer into small, clean squirt bottles.

Store in a cool place out of direct sunlight.

Remember to shake gently before each use.

Tea Tree Oil Sanitizer

Preparation Time: 10 minutes

Materials Needed:

Bowl and Spoon

Funnel

Squirt Bottles

Ingredients:

5 drops tea tree essential oil

1 tablespoon rubbing alcohol

½ tablespoons aloe vera gel

2 cups boiled and cooled water

Directions:

In a glass bowl, add the essential oil, tree oil and rubbing alcohol and stir to combine.

Add the aloe vera gel and mix until well combined.

Now, add the water and mix until well combined.

Through a funnel, pour the hand sanitizer into small, clean squirt bottles.

Store in a cool place out of direct sunlight.

Remember to shake gently before each use.

Natural Moisturizing Hand Sanitizer

Preparation Time: 20 minutes

Materials Needed: Bowls and Spoon - Funnel

Squirt Bottles

Ingredients: Vitamin E oil – ¼ teaspoon

Rubbing alcohol or high-proof vodka – 3 ounces

Tea tree essential oil – 30 drops

Sandalwood essential oil – 5 – 10 drops

Directions:

Add the Vitamin E oil and the essential oils to a small container or glass bowl and mix thoroughly.

Add alcohol to the bowl and mix again

Now add the aloe vera gel and blend well.

Transfer the mixture to clean colored bottles so that the essential oils in the recipe are not exposed to light

Shake gently before you use it.

The alcohol and Vitamin E oil helps to increase the shelf life of your sanitizer, for up to 6 months. To make your hand sanitizer spray with this recipe, replace the aloe vera gel with witch hazel.

Vetiver Oil Sanitizer

Preparation Time: 10 minutes

Materials Needed:

Bowl and Spoon

Funnel

Squirt Bottles

Ingredients: 15 drops vetiver essential oil

5 drops tea tree oil

1 tablespoon rubbing alcohol

½ tablespoons aloe vera gel

2 cups boiled and cooled water

Directions:

In a glass bowl, add the essential oil, tree oil and rubbing alcohol and stir to combine.

Add the aloe vera gel and mix until well combined.

Now, add the water and mix until well combined.

Through a funnel, pour the hand sanitizer into small, clean squirt bottles.

Store in a cool place out of direct sunlight.

Remember to shake gently before each use.

Cedarwood Oil Sanitizer

Preparation Time: 10 minutes

Materials Needed:

Bowl and Spoon

Funnel

Squirt Bottles

Ingredients: 5 drops cedarwood essential oil

5 drops tea tree oil

1 tablespoon rubbing alcohol

½ tablespoons aloe vera gel

2 cups boiled and cooled water

Directions:

In a glass bowl, add the essential oil, tree oil and rubbing alcohol and stir to combine.

Add the aloe vera gel and mix until well combined.

Now, add the water and mix until well combined.

Through a funnel, pour the hand sanitizer into small, clean squirt bottles.

Store in a cool place out of direct sunlight.

Remember to shake gently before each use.

Citrus Sanitizer Spray

Preparation Time: 20 minutes

Materials Needed: Bowl and Spoon - Funnel

Squirt Bottles

Ingredients:

5 Drops of Vitamin E oil

3 Tablespoons of Witch Hazel, Vodka, or Ever clear

5 Drops of Lemon Essential Oil

5 Drops of Orange Essential Oil

5 Drops of Tea Tree Essential Oil

Boiled water (Cooled down)

Directions:

Add water to the pan or pot that you will be using. Set this water to a boil for 5 to 10 minutes. After the boil is complete set the pan or pot of water aside to cool.

Add the vitamin E oil, choice of alcohol or witch hazel, and essential oils into the 2-ounce spray bottle. Close the top of the spray bottle and shake to combine all the ingredients into a uniform solution. Open the top of the bottle and pour the cooled down water that was boiled. Fill the bottle to the top and re-seal the bottle. Shake the spray bottle again for one final mix and your sanitizer spray is ready.

White Vinegar Sanitizer

Preparation Time: 10 minutes

Materials Needed:

Bowl and Spoon

Funnel

Squirt Bottles

Ingredients:

¼ cup white distilled vinegar (5% acidity)

½ cup distilled water

Directions:

In a glass bowl, add the vinegar and water and mix until well combined.

Through a funnel, pour the hand sanitizer into small, clean squirt bottles.

Store in a cool place out of direct sunlight.

Remember to shake gently before each use.

Apple Cider Vinegar Sanitizer

Preparation Time: 10 minutes

Materials Needed:

Bowl and Spoon

Funnel

Squirt Bottles

Ingredients:

¼ cup apple cider vinegar

½ cup aloe vera gel

Directions:

In a glass bowl, add the vinegar and aloe vera gel and mix until well combined.

Through a funnel, pour the hand sanitizer into small, clean squirt bottles.

Store in a cool place out of direct sunlight.

Remember to shake gently before each use.

Coconut Oil Sanitizer

Preparation Time: 10 minutes

Materials Needed:

Bowl and Spoon

Funnel

Squirt Bottles

Ingredients:

½ teaspoon sea salt

20 drops thieves young living oil

Distilled water, as required

2 teaspoons coconut oil

Directions:

In a small, clean glass squirt bottles, place the sea salt.

Now, place the thieves young living oil and set aside for about 5 minutes.

Place the enough distilled water, filling the bottle half the way.

Now, place the coconut oil into the bottle.

Shake the bottle until well combined.

Store in a cool place out of direct sunlight.

Remember to shake gently before each use.

Oils Sanitizer

Preparation Time: 10 minutes

Materials Needed: Bowl and Spoon – Funnel - Squirt Bottles

Ingredients:

½ teaspoon vitamin E oil

20 drops melaleuca essential oil

15 drops white fir essential oil

15 drops lemon essential oil

¼ cup alcohol-free witch hazel

½ cup pure aloe vera gel

¼ cup distilled water

Directions:

In a glass bowl, add the vitamin E oil, essential oils and witch hazel and stir to combine.

Add the aloe vera gel and mix until well combined.

Now, add the water and mix until well combined.

Through a funnel, pour the hand sanitizer into small, clean squirt bottles.

Store in a cool place out of direct sunlight.

Remember to shake gently before each use.

Nonalcoholic Hand Sanitizer

Preparation Time: 10 minutes

Materials Needed: Bowl and Spoon – Funnel - Squirt Bottles

Ingredients:

10 tbsp. of aloe vera gel

10 drops tea tree essential oil

20 drops lavender essential oil

10 drops orange essential oil

Directions:

First, prepare the aloe vera gel to make the antibacterial gel.

Put the gel in a bowl that is somewhat deep and also add the lavender essential oil and stir with a wooden or silicone spoon.

When it is well-integrated, then add the other two essential oils and stir well again.

Once you see the ingredients well integrated, pour the mixture into a pot in which you are going to store the antibacterial. We recommend that you have a dispenser and that it closes well. You can store it in several smaller boats so you can easily carry one with you.

Since it does not have alcohol, if you want this gel to be well preserved, we recommend that you use a dark bottle or, at least, do not leave it exposed to light regularly, since it would not hold as well preserved.

Lemon-mint Essential Oil Hand Wash

Preparation Time: 15 minutes

Materials Needed:

Bowl and Spoon

Funnel

Squirt Bottles

Ingredients:

¾ cup of water

¼ cup of castile soap

20 drops of lemon-mint essential oil

Soap dispenser

Directions:

Wash and rinse out any oil soap dispenser

Pour ¾ cups of water into the dispenser

Add ¼ cups of castile soap

Add 20 drops of lemon-mint oil to the mixture

Place the dispenser lid and shake well.

Witch Hazel Sanitizer

Preparation Time: 15 minutes

Materials Needed: Bowl and Spoon

Funnel

Squirt Bottles

Ingredients:

1 tbsp. of witch hazel

10 drops essential oil

9 tbsp. of pure aloe vera

20 drops tea tree oil

Dosing container

Mixing bowl

Funnel (optional).

Directions:

Place the witch hazel in a bowl, and, little by little, we add one by one the rest of the ingredients.

Once this is ready, remove with a spoon so that all the oils are well integrated. The gel should be thick and viscous.

Put the gel in the prepared dosing container. If the nozzle is tiny, use a funnel so that the mixture does not spill.

Citrus Hand Sanitizer

Preparation Time: 15 minutes

Materials Needed: Bowl and Spoon

Funnel

Squirt Bottles

Ingredients:

6 tbsp. (90 ml. / 3 fl. oz.) isopropyl alcohol (99% rubbing alcohol)

2 tbsp. (30 ml. / 1 fl. oz.) aloe vera gel

8 drops vitamin E oil

5 drops tea tree essential oil

5 drops lemon essential oil

5 drops lime essential oil

distilled water

Directions:

Put the alcohol, aloe vera gel, and vitamin E oil into a small jar. Gently mix, or put on the lid and swirl the ingredients together. Add the essential oils a few drops at a time, slowly swirling the jar or stirring. Add a bit of distilled water to achieve your desired consistency, put the lid on the jar and vigorously shake it to combine all the ingredients. Store in a container of your choice.

Alcoholic Antibacterial Sanitizer

Preparation Time: 10 minutes

Materials Needed: Bowl and Spoon

Funnel

Squirt Bottles

Ingredients:

20 ml witch hazel

70 ml 96% ethyl alcohol/ethanol

¼ tbsp. of vegetable glycerin

20 drops eucalyptus/rosemary essential oil

Directions:

Buy or prepare witch hazel water; you can make it as a cold infusion, leaving some flowers and leaves to rest for several hours and then removing the remains.

In the measuring container in which you are going to store the final homemade disinfectant gel, add the witch hazel water, the alcohol, and the prepared vegetable glycerin.

Mix well until the ingredients are integrated and add the drops of the essential oil you have chosen.

Stir well again, and when you see a homogeneous mixture, you will have your natural antibacterial gel ready!

Lime Oil Sanitizer

Preparation Time: 10 minutes

Materials Needed: Bowl and Spoon

Funnel

Squirt Bottles

Ingredients:

5 drops lime essential oil

5 drops tea tree oil

1 tablespoon rubbing alcohol

½ tablespoons aloe vera gel

2 cups boiled and cooled water

Directions:

In a glass bowl, add the essential oil, tree oil and rubbing alcohol and stir to combine.

Add the aloe vera gel and mix until well combined.

Now, add the water and mix until well combined.

Through a funnel, pour the hand sanitizer into small, clean squirt bottles.

Store in a cool place out of direct sunlight.

Remember to shake gently before each use.

Lemon Oil Sanitizer

Preparation Time: 10 minutes

Materials Needed: Bowl and Spoon

Funnel

Squirt Bottles

Ingredients:

5 drops lemon essential oil

5 drops tea tree oil

1 tablespoon rubbing alcohol

½ tablespoons aloe vera gel

2 cups boiled and cooled water

Directions:

In a glass bowl, add the essential oil, tree oil and rubbing alcohol and stir to combine.

Add the aloe vera gel and mix until well combined.

Now, add the water and mix until well combined.

Through a funnel, pour the hand sanitizer into small, clean squirt bottles.

Store in a cool place out of direct sunlight.

Remember to shake gently before each use.

Tea Tree Hand Sanitizer Spray

Preparation Time: 20 minutes

Materials Needed:

Bowl and Spoon

Funnel

Squirt Bottles

Ingredients:

Aloe vera gel – 6 Tbsp.

91% Isopropyl rubbing alcohol – 4 Tbsp.

Tea tree oil – 20 drops

Directions:

Mix all your ingredients in a bowl, then transfer to a spray bottle.

Shake well before you use to get the essential oils evenly distributed.

Lemon Oil Hand Sanitizer Spray

Preparation Time: 20 minutes

Materials Needed:

Bowl and Spoon

Funnel

Squirt Bottles

Ingredients:

Distilled water

Tea tree essential oil – 5 drops

Lemon essential oil – 5 drops

Rubbing alcohol – 2 Tbsp.

A squirt of aloe vera gel

Directions:

Add the rubbing alcohol, essential oils, and the aloe vera gel into a spray bottle

Shake, then fill the rest of the bottle with your water and shake again.

Your spray is ready for use.

Vitamin E Oil Spray

Preparation Time: 10 minutes

Materials Needed:

Bowl and Spoon

Funnel

Squirt Bottles

Ingredients:

Vitamin B oil 5drops

Tea tree oil - 5 drops

Aloe vera gel - 3 tablespoons

Dispenser tube

Water filtered - 2 cups

Directions:

Mix all the ingredients together. Then add water and shake vigorously, at this point let it rest a bit. Now we are ready to use it.

Pure Aloe Vera Spray

Preparation Time: 10 minutes

Materials Needed:

Bowl and Spoon

Funnel

Squirt Bottles

Ingredients:

Lavender essential oil - 5 drops

Tea tree oil - 5 drops

Pure aloe vera gel - 8 ounces

Hazel extract - 1 tablespoon

Vitamin E e oil - ¼ teaspoons

Directions:

Mix the lavender oil and vitamin e oil together in a bowl and while stirring it, add the hazel extract along with the tea tree oil. When it is all blended completely, add the aloe vera gel into it. Pour it in a bottle and then mix well every time you want to use it. Preferably, it should be the spray bottle.

Using Peppermint Essential Oil

Preparation Time: 15 minutes

Materials Needed:

Bowl and Spoon

Funnel

Squirt Bottles

Ingredients:

2/3 cup of the proof grain alcohol

1/3 cup of the aloe vera gel (make sure that it does not have any additives)

Eight drops of the essential oil, (peppermint)

Plastic container, funnel, spoon and the mixing bowl

Directions:

Pour all the ingredients in the pan and start mixing them using the spoon. Make sure that the mixture is smooth. If you want to make the solution even thicker, you can add another spoon of the aloe vera in it. Similarly, if you want the mixture to be thin, add another spoon of the alcohol in it.

Now add the essential oil in the mixture; in this case, we are using peppermint oil. You can use other essential oils as well based on your choices. The addition of the essential oil is mainly for the smell. When you add the peppermint oil, check the scent, if you don't like it, try adding some more drops of it.

The other options for the essential oils include clove, lavender, and cinnamon. These all have the antiseptic properties in it. There are some different scents as well, which can be used in the mixture; you can use grapefruit, passion fruit, and the lemon for improving the smell of the hand sanitizers.

Add the mixture into the container. You can add it in a small bottle as well and carry it anywhere with you. If you are making it in a higher quantity, you can save it in a jar at your home.

Capitolo 9 : DIY Hand Sanitizer Disinfectant Wipes for Hands and Surfaces

One major benefit of making disinfectant wipes at home rather than buying them is that commercial hand wipes contain harmful toxins like triclosan and phthalates. Triclosan is an antibacterial and antifungal agent used in soap, deodorants, sanitizers and more. It has been linked to severe concerns like endocrine disruption, eye and skin irritation and organ toxicity. Phthalates are used as solvents and are also used to make plastic flexible. Phthalates has been linked to low sperm count, disruption of endocrine system and liver cancer among other things.

Making your own hand wipes will protect you from the harmful effects of these nasty chemicals they add to commercial wipes, at a cheaper cost.

Some of the recipes below contain alcohol while others do not so you can pick the one that suits your need.

To make your homemade hand wipes, you will need:

- **Dry wipes -** you can order these on Amazon or buy from a store near you. You can also use small wash cloths and wash them after every use.

- **Essential oils**- you can use whichever one that you like. I prefer tea tree oil and tangerine oil. Tea tree oil is a natural antibacterial and is excellent for the skin, while tangerine oil has a lovely citrus scent that will leave your wipes with a fresh and clean aroma.

- **Liquid soap**- I use castile soap because it contains olive oil which is gentle on the skin and does not foam up or leave sticky residue on your skin like other types of soap do. Make sure your soap is unscented so that it does not mix with the smell of the essential oils.

- **Distilled water**- you can make it by boiling your tap water.

- **Airtight container**- this is to use as storage for your wipes once they are ready. A Tupperware container or a Ziploc bad will do.

- Measuring cup and spoon

Sweet Orange Natural Sanitizing Wipes

Preparation Time: 15 minutes

Materials Needed:

Wipes/ Reusable Towels

Bottle or Container

Ingredients

50 dry wipes

4 drops, orange essential oil

3 drops, tea tree oil

12 oz. distilled water

½ teaspoon castile soap

Measuring cup and spoon

Directions:

Wash your hands before you start to prevent contamination of the wipes

Place wipes in a container with a tight lid so they remain fresh.

To get the liquid formula ready, mix the distilled water, essential oils and castile soap in a bowl.

Gently pour the mixture over the wipes while lifting sections of the stack of wipes to allow the mixture to soak through the entire stack.

When you finish pouring the mixture, use both fists to press down on the soaps to further help the mixture soak into the wipes. Repeat until the wipes are well saturated with the mixture.

These wipes should last between 2-3 weeks since they do not have any preservatives in them.

Natural Disinfectant Wipes

Preparation Time: 10 minutes

Materials Needed: Wipes/ Reusable Towels

Bottle or Container

Ingredients: 1 ½ cups, 100 proof vodka.

½ cup, white distilled vinegar (or more alcohol)

50-60 drops, tea tree essential oil

Directions:

Place the wipes/reusable towels in a container

Pour vodka into a bottle followed by the tea tree oil

Shake bottle to combine the vodka and oils

Add the vinegar and shake again

Pour the mixture over the wipes in the container until all wipes are well saturated. If using dry wipes, you may need to double up the recipe.

Your wipes are ready to use!

Simply re-wet the disinfecting towels with the same solution whenever they start to dry out.

Note: The essential oil works as an antibacterial ingredient. Hydrogen peroxide can also work as a disinfectant when used straight and not diluted or mixed with other things. Do not mix with vinegar!

Alcohol-free wipes

Preparation Time: 15 minutes

Materials Needed:

Wipes/ Reusable Towels

Bottle or Container

Ingredients: 20 paper towels - ¼ cup, witch hazel

¼ cup, aloe vera gel

¼ cup filtered water

10 drops, tea tree oil

10 drops, peppermint essential oil

1 tbsp., vegetable glycerin

1 tbsp., apple cider vinegar

Directions:

Mix all your ingredients in a large bowl

Cut paper towels in half or buy those that come in different sizes.

Roll up the towels and dip them in the mixture until they are well saturated.

Lastly, transfer the towels into a Ziploc bag or reusable baby wipe container for storage.

Use as needed.

Vinegar Based Disinfectant Wipes

Preparation Time: 10 minutes

Materials Needed: Wipes/ Reusable Towels

Jar or Container

Bowl and spoon

Ingredients:

¾ Cup Boiled water (Cooled Down)

¾ Cup Distilled Vinegar

15 Drops Lemon Essential Oil

8 Drops Lavender Essential Oil

4 Drops Bergamot Essential Oil

Directions:

Add water to the pot or pan. Bring it to a boil on a stovetop for 5 to 10 minutes. After this set the water aside to cool. This will be the water that is used in the solution in the recipe.

Cut the washcloths up into the size desired. Generally, these are cut in half. Place them into the mason jar or other container. Add the water, essential oils, and vinegar to a bowl. Mix these until the solution becomes uniform. Add the solution to the jar that contains the wipes. Close the lid of the jar and let the wipes soak. Store until they need to be used.

Gel Aloe Hand Wipe

Preparation Time: 15 minutes

Materials Needed: Wipes/ Reusable Towels - Jar or Container

Bowl and spoon

Ingredients: Small reusable towels that can be washed, body wipes, dry wipes or baby wipes

Glass or plastic container with a lid like a zip-top bag or a Tupperware container

Gel aloe – 2 tablespoons

Hot water – 1 cup

70% rubbing alcohol – 4 tablespoons

A mixing bowl or cup

Mixing spoon

Directions: Place the wipes/ reusable towels into a container.

Mix the rubbing alcohol, aloe gel, and hot water in a bowl until well mixed. Pour the mixture over the wipes in the container until all the wipes are well saturated. You may need to double up the recipe if using dry wipes. And your wipe is ready!

Re-wet the sanitizing towels with the same solution whenever they dry out.

DIY Natural Hand Wipes

Preparation Time: 15 minutes

Materials Needed: Wipes/ Reusable Towels - Jar or Container

Bowl and spoon

Ingredients: Dry wipes - 50 - Tea Tree Essential oils – 3 drops

Orange Essential oils – 4 drops

Distilled water – 12 oz (You can boil your water as an alternative to distilled water.)

Castile soap – ½ teaspoon - Measuring cup and spoon

Directions: Wash your hands before you begin to reduce the amount of contamination in the wipe.

Place the wipes in a Tupperware-type container that has a tight lid to keep them fresh.

Now get your liquid formula ready. Feel free to add or remove from this recipe. Mix the essential oils, castile soap, and the distilled water.

Now pour the liquid over the wipes little by little. Lift sections of your stack so that the liquid can soak through the entire stack. After you have emptied the liquid, use both fists to press down on the top of the wipe to help the liquid soak into the wipes. Repeat this until the liquid is well saturated.

These wipes do not have preservatives in them, and so, they should last for two to three weeks.

Alcohol-Free Hand Wipes

Preparation Time: 15 minutes

Materials Needed: Wipes/ Reusable Towels - Jar or Container

Bowl and spoon

Ziploc Bag

Ingredients: Witch hazel - 1/4 cup

Filtered water - 1/4 cup

Aloe vera gel - 1/4 cup

Apple cider vinegar - 1 tbsp

Vegetable glycerin - 1 tbsp

Peppermint essential oil – 10 drops

Tea tree oil – 10 drops

Paper towel - 20

Directions:

Mix all the ingredients in a large bowl.

Cut the paper towels in half or purchase the one that comes in different sizes.

Roll the paper towels and dip in the mixture until well saturated.

Then transfer the towel into a leftover baby wipe container or Ziploc bag.

Tangerine Oil Hand Wipes

Preparation Time: 15 minutes

Materials Needed: Wipes/ Reusable Towels

Jar or Container

Bowl and spoon

Ziploc Bag

Ingredients:

Aloe vera gel - ½ cup

Filtered water - ¼ cup

Vodka or rubbing alcohol - ¼ cup

Witch hazel - 1 tbsp

Tea tree essential oil – 10 drops

Tangerine essential oil – 10 drops

Directions:

Mix all the ingredients in a large bowl.

Cut the paper towels in half or purchase the one that comes in different sizes.

Roll the paper towels and dip in the mixture until well saturated.

Then transfer the towel into a leftover baby wipe container or Ziploc bag.

Homemade Antibacterial Wipes

Preparation Time: 10 minutes

Materials Needed: Wipes/ Reusable Towels - Jar or Container

Bowl and spoon - Ziploc Bag

This wipe is active and will not dry your skin even with repeated use. Thanks to the lotion in the recipe.

Ingredients: Homemade lotion – 16 oz. (see recipe down)

Lemon essential oil - 5 drops - Orange essential oil – 10 drops

Heavy-duty paper towels - Rubbing alcohol – 16 oz.

Directions:

Place the essential oils, rubbing alcohol and lotion in a container or Ziploc bag. Knead the ingredients together to get them well mixed.

If using big paper towels, cut them into 3 pieces (or to a size that suits you).

Transfer the pieces of the paper towel to another container then pour the liquid over the sheets.

Allow to sit for a minimum of 30 minutes to get the towels well soaked in the liquid. You can turn the container upside down to achieve this.

Add more paper towels if the towels are too wet for you.

Divide the wipes into separate Ziploc bags and place them in different strategic locations like your car, in the kitchen, and your handbag.

DIY Cleaning Wipes Recipe

Preparation Time: 15 minutes

Materials Needed:

1-pound espresso canister with plastic top

Scissors

Needle

Spray paint

Sharp blade

Paper towel roll

Ingredients:

10 drops basic oil

1 tsp. fluid dish cleanser

¼ tsp. scouring liquor

¼ cup of water

½ cup vinegar

Directions:

With a blade, cut the paper towels down the middle.

Squish them into the painted can.

Mix the water, liquor, dish cleanser, scarcely any drops of fundamental oil, and vinegar in a bowl.

Slowly pour the fluid over the paper towels.

Saturate them. At that point delicately evacuate the cardboard community and pull a paper towel from the inside.

Cut a 1 ½ inch distance across hovering in the focal point of the plastic cover.

Pass a touch of the paper towel through the gap and spread the can with the cover.

You can include a couple of drops of water into the canister to keep the wipes sodden.

Use!

DIY Cleaning Wipes Recipe 2

Preparation Time: 15 minutes

Materials Needed:

Bowl and Spoon

Paper Towels

Ingredients:

2 cups warm water

1 cup scouring liquor (in any event 70% liquor focus)

1 tbsp. dish cleanser

Directions:

Mix the fixings well.

Add this blend to a large portion of a move of paper towels in a Tupperware box.

DIY Disinfectant Wipes Recipe

Preparation Time: 15 minutes

Materials Needed:

1 perfect, old shirt (slice up to be utilized as wipes)

Scissors

An enormous container

Ingredients:

1 cup sifted or refined water

½ cup of vinegar

¼ cup scouring liquor (70% liquor fixation at any rate)

1 tsp. fluid Castile cleanser

8 to 12 drops of basic oils from 2 of the accompanying: lavender, tea tree, germ warrior, lemon, and any sort of citrus

Directions:

Add all the fluid fixings together in the container and blend.

Add wipes in the container and permit them to ingest the fluid. Spread the pot and shake well.

The wipes ought to be altogether clammy yet not sopping. Include more water if necessary.

Secure the cover firmly and store it in a cool, dry spot.

DIY Antibacterial Hand Wipes Recipe

Preparation Time: 15 minutes

Materials Needed:

30 paper towels cut down the middle

Airtight holder for capacity

Ingredients:

1 ¼ cup isopropyl liquor (70% or more)

1 tbsp. hydrogen peroxide

1 tsp. glycerin

¼ cup of refined water

Directions:

Mix the fixings in a bowl with a whisk.

In a spotless stockpiling holder, stack up paper towels.

Pour the fluid blend over the paper towels.

Close the top and shake well.

Make sure all the paper towels get doused well.

Shake well before each utilization.

Ideas on How to Customize Your Wipes

Add more or less liquid depending on if you like your wipes barely moist or super wet.

Cut the wipes in quarters or half to give you different sizes.

Feel free to experiment with different essential oils. Here are some options for you to try:

Lavender Oil: to fight germs and for a great scent.

Lemon oil: has a lovely fresh scent

Thieves oil/ germ fighter: several essential oil providers carry this oil. I will advise you to use this, particularly when sickness or disease is going around like strep or stomach bug.

Thyme, Clove, Rosemary, and Cinnamon: these oils have an overpowering smell, so you need to be careful how you mix them.

Calendula oil: this oil has antifungal, antibacterial, and anti-inflammatory properties that help in soothing eczema and/ or heal wounds.

Capitolo 10 : Alcohol-free and Alternative Hand Sanitizer Recipes

Safe Recipes for Kids

Preparation time: 10 minutes

Ingredients:

1/4 cup of aloe vera gel

20 drops of Germ Destroyer EO (This is kid friendly or safe)

Instructions:

Mix all ingredients together and store in a silicone tube container.

Use as needed to naturally kill 99.9% germs from hands.

On Guard Oil Sanitizer

Preparation time: 10 minutes

Ingredients:

20 drop dōTERRAon Guard EO

1 tablespoon aloe vera gel

Boiled and cooled water, as required

Instructions:

In a small, clean squirt bottle, place the oil and aloe vera gel.

Now, fill the remaining bottle with water.

Shake the bottle until well combined.

Store in a cool place out of direct sunlight.

Remember to shake lightly before using.

Alcohol-Free Witch Hazel Sanitizer

Preparation time: 10 minutes

Ingredients:

¼ teaspoon Vitamin E oil

30 drops tea tree oil

1 tablespoon alcohol-free witch hazel

1 tablespoon aloe vera gel

Instructions:

In a glass bowl, add the Vitamin E oil, tree oil and witch hazel and stir to combine.

Add the aloe vera gel and mix until well combined.

Through a funnel, pour the hand sanitizer into small, clean squirt bottles.

Store in a cool place out of direct sunlight.

Remember to shake lightly before using.

Germ Destroyer Oil Sanitizer

Preparation time: 10 minutes

Ingredients:

20 drops germ destroyer EO

¼ cup aloe vera gel

Instructions:

In a glass bowl, add the EO and aloe vera gel and mix until well combined.

Through a funnel, pour the hand sanitizer into small, clean squirt bottles.

Store in a cool place out of direct sunlight.

Remember to shake lightly before using.

Vitamin E Oil Sanitizer

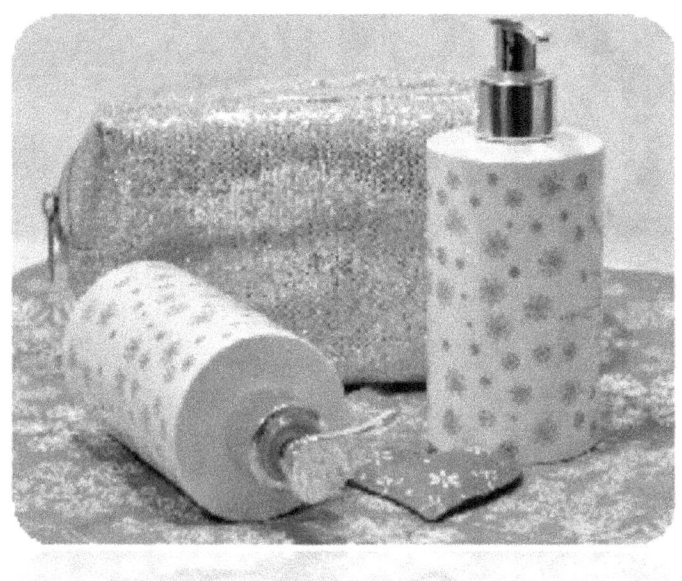

Preparation time: 10 minutes

Ingredients:

5 drops Vitamin E oil

5 drops tea tree oil

3 tablespoons aloe vera gel

2 cups boiled and cooled water

Instructions:

In a glass bowl, add the Vitamin E oil and tree oil and stir to combine.

Add the aloe vera gel and mix until well combined.

Now, add the water and mix until well combined.

Through a funnel, pour the hand sanitizer into small, clean squirt bottles.

Store in a cool place out of direct sunlight.

Remember to shake lightly before using.

White Vinegar Sanitizer

Preparation time: 10 minutes

Ingredients: ¼ cup white distilled vinegar (5% acidity)

½ cup distilled water

Instructions:

In a glass bowl, add the vinegar and water and mix until well combined.

Through a funnel, pour the hand sanitizer into small, clean squirt bottles.

Store in a cool place out of direct sunlight.

Remember to shake lightly before using.

Apple Cider Vinegar Sanitizer

Preparation time: 10 minutes

Ingredients:

¼ cup apple cider vinegar

½ cup aloe vera gel

Instructions:

In a glass bowl, add the vinegar and aloe vera gel and mix until well combined.

Through a funnel, pour the hand sanitizer into small, clean squirt bottles.

Store in a cool place out of direct sunlight.

Remember to shake lightly before using.

4 Oils Sanitizer

Preparation time: 10 minutes

Ingredients:

½ teaspoon vitamin E oil

20 drops melaleuca EO

15 drops white fir EO

15 drops lemon EO

¼ cup alcohol-free witch hazel

½ cup pure aloe vera gel

¼ cup distilled water

Instructions:

In a glass bowl, add the vitamin E oil, EOs and witch hazel and stir to combine.

Add the aloe vera gel and mix until well combined.

Now, add the water and mix until well combined.

Through a funnel, pour the hand sanitizer into small, clean squirt bottles.

Store in a cool place out of direct sunlight.

Remember to shake lightly before using.

5 Oils Sanitizer

Preparation time: 10 minutes

Ingredients:

20 drops orange EO

10 drops lavender EO

10 drops cinnamon EO

5 drops rosemary EO

5 drops clove EO

¼ cup aloe vera gel

Instructions:

In a glass bowl, add all the EOs and stir to combine.

Add the aloe vera gel and mix until well combined.

Through a funnel, pour the hand sanitizer into small, clean squirt bottles.

Store in a cool place out of direct sunlight.

Remember to shake lightly before using.

Castile Soap & tea Tree Oil Sanitizer

Preparation time: 10 minutes

Ingredients:

10 drops tea tree EO

1 teaspoon castile soap

6 ounces boiled and cooled water

Instructions:

In a glass bowl, add the EO and castile soap and stir to combine.

Now, add the water and mix until well combined.

Through a funnel, pour the hand sanitizer into small, clean squirt bottles.

Store in a cool place out of direct sunlight.

Remember to shake lightly before using.

Capitolo 11 : How to Boost Your Immune System

After learning the facts about your immune system, it is equally important to know how to maintain and promote its health. Keep in mind that anything that damages cells or tissues can damage the immune system. The steps below will help you boost your immune system.

Step #1—Acquire a positive way of thinking

Believe it or not, thinking positively in any given situation is one definite way to boost your immune system. This is due to the fact that when you think positively, your brain commands the body to respond accordingly. It's your brain that stimulates your hormones to respond. It produces physical manifestations in your body that can influence your immune system. The brain is a powerful tool that controls all your body's systems, so feed it only with positive thoughts and good "food".

A positive way of thinking reduces stress and prevents the increased secretion of the stress hormone glucocorticoids. How reduction of stress can boost your immune system is presented in step #2.

Step #2—Cope with stress effectively

This is connected to your being an optimist. You will most likely agree that when you think positively, you will feel less stressed, because you will worry less. Worrying less will prevent the secretion of hormones such as epinephrine and norepinephrine that can elevate your blood pressure and exert undue pressure on your organs and on your immune system.

Stress also increases the secretion of your glucocorticoids that can affect the thymus which produces your lymphocytes. Glucocorticoid is a stress hormone produced by the adrenal glands that plays a detrimental role in the immune system. It inhibits vital substances such as, interleukins and cytokines. These two substances are vital in the activity of white blood cells—the primary cells involved in your immune response.

Learn how to cope with stress and how to relax daily. There are numerous techniques you can employ to relax yourself. Yoga, meditation and breathing exercises are the most common options.

Set aside time every day just to sit and relax in order to free yourself of stress. Breathing in and out deeply for a few minutes can relax you. Doing some muscle stretches for a few minutes can also do the trick.

Step #3—Eat more fruits and vegetables

Your immune system thrives on the cells that can properly perform their functions. These cells rely on your diet to stay strong and healthy. Studies have established that fruits and vegetables are beneficial to a person's health. This is because they are rich in essential nutrients that the body needs, sufficient fiber for gut health, and vitamins needed for cells, tissues and organs' development and growth.

Fruits, especially citrus fruits, and vegetables such as mushrooms and green leafy vegetables can also provide vitamins A, B, C, D, and E that your immune system needs. They contain chlorophyll and anti-oxidants that help cells stay healthy. They can also provide the minerals that your body needs such as potassium, magnesium, chloride, sodium, calcium and phosphorus.

Step #4—Don't drink alcohol

Your immune system depends significantly on the proper function of your cells, which is damaged by alcohol. When these body cells are impaired, your immune system is damaged too. Acetaldehyde, one of the end products of alcohol metabolism, has been found to cause liver cirrhosis. This toxic substance slowly kills cells and renders them keratinized or dead. It's like you're committing suicide slowly and deliberately.

Aside from that, alcohol is a central nerve depressant that can diminish the normal function of your body's systems. This can lead to dysfunctions in your whole body including your immune system. You wouldn't want to keep drinking alcohol if you value your body and your health.

Step #5—Exercise daily

You may have read this advice several times, and may even think it's overrated. The fact remains, that you can never run away from exercise if you want to boost your immune system. Exercise is one of the inevitable pillars of good health. When you exercise, your blood circulation improves and your cells are adequately nourished. Remember that your white blood cells are the major cells involved in your immune system, hence if they are properly nourished, they can function effectively. Also, when you exercise, you sweat a lot. Sweating is one action of the immune system to get rid of microbes and toxic substances from your body. Furthermore, exercise can prevent obesity and keep you at your ideal weight. Sweat it out and help your immune system clean up your body. Exercise those muscles daily and let the blood flow smoothly in your blood vessels throughout your body.

Walk, jog, cycle, do aerobics or engage in sports to exercise those muscles and strengthen your defenses. It doesn't matter what type of exercise you engage in as long as you flex those muscles and work up a sweat. This can take from 30 minutes to one hour daily.

Step #6—Get enough sleep

It's when you sleep that some important substances and hormones are released sufficiently. Examples of these are Growth Hormone (GH) and Growth Hormone Releasing Hormone (GHRH). These hormones are important aspects in the growth of your cells and tissues. Anything that impedes the growth of cells will always impede the development of your immune system too.

Outside of your immune system, lack of sleep has many detrimental effects that can be fatal. Your brain is impaired too, affecting the normal functions of your body systems. Children need 8 to 10 hours sleep, while adults need at least 7 to 8 hours of sleep.

Step #7—Avoid bad fats, excess sugar and excess salt

Bad fats come from meat fat and dairy products, while good fats come from fruits and vegetables. Fats can cause various diseases such as, cardiac and liver disease. Bad fats can also weaken your immune system.

Too much sugar and salt can also damage your cells and tissues, and thereby, your immune system. Sugar in blood comes from carbohydrates such as, rice, pasta and bread, so don't overeat and make yourself sick. Salt comes from your plain table salt and is typically present in high levels in processed food. Taking too much salt can weaken your immune system because the water-electrolyte balance will not be maintained.

Step #8—Avoid illicit drugs

Drugs of abuse attack the cells of your body and destroy them. Take note that your major immunity players are your WBC, lymphocytes, neutrophils and eosinophils, which are all blood cells. Therefore, if these are all attacked by the components of your illicit drugs, then your immune system will be weakened significantly. Illicit drugs can affect your brain too and can harm your central nervous system. Plus—you risk jail time by using these addictive drugs. So, stay away from them!

Step #9—Don't smoke or drink too much coffee

The nicotine in cigarettes is harmful to blood cells. In fact, it destroys your respiratory cells and can cause lung cancer and other lung diseases. It can do the same damage to the cells of your immune system.

In the same manner that nicotine is bad for you, coffee can only cause harm in the long term. The caffeine in coffee can wake you up because it stimulates your hormones, but too much of it can have unhealthy repercussions. Both nicotine and caffeine tend to be addictive so these substances must be avoided.

Step #10—Take probiotics

A healthy gut will boost your immune system, so consume probiotics that contain healthy bacteria for your stomach. These bacteria (lactobacilli) are part of the normal flora of your stomach. They drive out the pathogenic microbes. Taking probiotics will help maintain the balance of the good bacteria inside your gut, consequently resulting in a better performing immune system. Probiotics is typically found in yogurt and other special beverages.

Step #11—Add more protein in your diet

Your antibodies are protein in nature, so protein in your diet can help boost your immune system. In addition, the amino acids coming from your protein diet are the building blocks of the growth and development of your cells. Sans these amino acids, you can't grow a single cell in your body. Examples of proteins are lean meat, soya beans, fish and egg white.

Step #12—Maintain a healthy social life

Scientists have confirmed that being able to live a happy social life, and being able to develop meaningful relationships can boost your immune system. This stems from the fact that when you have a healthy social life you tend to be happier and less stressed. With these positive emotions, your immune system is given a boost because your cells are produced properly without any interruptions from stress and unhappiness.

So, when you ask the question: how can these feelings affect your immune system? Remember that all emotions are sent to your brain and the brain reacts to manage them by stimulating the glands to produce specific hormones.

Studies also established that T cell functions have increased in people who have had successful relationships. Likewise, the antibody, IgG, increases when people socialize more. IgG fights off infections together with the other immunoglobulins.

Capitolo 12 : Secrets to Protect Yourself Against Current Outbreaks and Neutralize Pandemics

Some useful tips to avoid any danger of contagion have been provided by the WHO, World Health Organization.

The cleaning of the rooms, of course, must be preceded by good practices on hygiene rules, first of all wash your hands often. Among the behaviors to be adopted are: Leave clothes and shoes outside the home, or at least get rid of the clothes worn to go out already at the entrance of the home. Especially for those who continue to go to work: everything that comes from outside - including clothes - and that could be contaminated must, in some way, be defused.

Leading a healthy life is and should be the top most priority for every person. Being on a sick bed makes us realize how lucky being healthy is, and how grateful we should be for every moment we spend disease free.

The world that we are living in today is becoming increasingly dangerous. The reason is not just the political turmoil that every country is in, but also the increasing rate of natural calamities that we are facing.

With the start of the year 2020, we saw the world changing before our very eyes. Climate change was the real threat following us for the last few years, the fear of losing our planet to increasingly hazardous effects of carbon emissions.

If this wasn't enough, Coronavirus pandemic hit us like it has never before. Considered and called out for being 'just a flu' for the first few days that it emerged, this disease changed its course and took everyone by surprise. Starting from China, it spread on to become a global pandemic, engulfing giant countries like the US. In the midst of all the panic that ensued following the spread of Covid-19, human kind suffered from crisis after crisis. From shortage of toilet papers and hand sanitizers to basic food necessities, we saw it all.

When it became increasingly clear that the shortage of these hygiene products was inevitable and the hikes in their prices in some countries made it impossible for a common man to buy them, we turned to something else. We started trying to make soaps and hand sanitizers at home. This also aims at helping you with the very same thing. It is very important to be calm and not panic while we fight together with these viruses that are attacking us so frequently.

There are some healthcare safety tips that we have combined here to help you stay safe from a very large number of diseases. These are simple yet effective strategies to stay safe from the dangers that we are facing these days.

How to prevent yourself from getting sick:

Keep your hands clean

Wash, wash and wash

This has been our mantra from the very start. No matter what else you do to keep yourself safe from disease, do not forget that handwashing should be your number one priority. Handwashing alone can help save you from many illnesses. Our hands consciously and unconsciously get in contact with many contaminated surfaces throughout the day, and when these hands touch the mucus membranes of the body, bacteria and viruses get a free pass inside you.

If you do not have access to clean water and soap everywhere, an alcohol based hand sanitizer can be your next best friend. Washing hands can literally save lives.

Stay at home when you are sick

Another important thing to keep in mind is that there are countless contagious diseases, even a simple cold or flu, that can spread if you go out unnecessarily while you are sick. Even in the pandemic like Covid-19, the best advice that the health experts gave was to self-isolate in case you feel sick. By staying at home, you can prevent spreading illnesses to other people. In the recent Covid-19 scenario, using health measures and self-quarantine itself helped a lot and kept the hospitals from getting overwhelmingly full.

Eat green vegetables

A lot of people don't like eating vegetables, especially the boring greens. Well, this time you should keep in mind that the green vegetables are full of nutritious juices and a wide variety of vitamins. Taking plenty of vitamins can help keep you away from many diseases. It fortifies your immune system and helps you in fighting viral infections specifically.

Get proper sleep

We cannot stress more on how important sleep is to keep your body healthy and fit. Sleep essentially restores your body and makes you a new person every morning you wake up. Sleep replenishes your body and reinvigorates it. Another important thing to keep in mind is that an adequate amount of sleep helps you in fighting off microbes and helps in building resistance against viral attacks.

Get vaccinated!

Remember that the only thing that is going to save you from many fatal diseases is a dose of vaccine. Vaccine does not damage your body, and no, it does not give you more diseases. In simple words, it is merely a harmless form of microbes that is injected into your body so that the body can recognize it and build immunity. So, the next time that microbe attacks, your body will already know how to fight against it and will not be taken by surprise.

Take proper nutrition

Your body is going to build from the food you eat. If you eat healthy, your mind and body stays healthy, and if you don't, you get sick. There are many foods that can specifically help in building your immunity. We have made a list of a few foods to get you started:

- Citrus fruits: Citrus fruits contain a large amount of vitamin C. Vitamin C is our savior in fighting against diseases, specifically viral illness. It helps in building your immunity by increasing the number of white blood cells in the body. These include lemons, oranges, grapefruit.

- Spinach: Ever wondered why the health experts always advise you to eat green veggies like spinach regularly? It is because spinach is a wonderous vegetable. It is not only rich in vitamin C but also provides your body with a wide variety of antioxidants to keep you healthy

- Sunflower seeds: Not widely eaten, but sunflower seeds are packed with nutrients. The most important nutrient in these seeds is Vitamin E. Like vitamin C, vitamin E also helps to some extent in building your immunity. Vitamin E also acts as an antioxidant.

Let's get back to hand hygiene as it is the single most important factor in prevention of illnesses.

Hand sanitizers play a very important part in maintenance of hygiene. Water and soap are not accessible everywhere and that is why hand sanitizers can help ward off bacteria and viruses for some time. Like every other product, the efficacy of hand sanitizers also depend on its adequate usage. It is very important to know how to properly use these products and what safety concerns should be kept in mind while using them

Here we will give you a quick summary on what to avoid and keep in mind while using hand sanitizers, whether commercially produced or handmade.

What to keep in mind while using hand sanitizers:

- Hand sanitizers, while being very important for hygiene, do not substitute hand washing. These cannot be used on your hands if there is visible dirt on it. In these cases, you must wash your hands first to remove the dirt.

- It is important to know the composition of the products that you are using. Products that contain large quantities of chemicals will do more harm than good.

- Make sure that you are not using a large quantity of essential oils in your homemade preparations. Although essential oils give a soothing effect to the skin, excessive use is not advised.

- Try to test a small quantity of whichever product you use on a small patch of skin first. Every person's skin is different and while one product is suitable for one skin, it might not be good for another person. In people that have sensitive skin type, using harsh chemicals or excessive drying of skin produces adverse reactions and may cause

- damage. It is important to report to a healthcare professional if you are having any serious symptoms

- Keep these products out of the reach of children as many of them might contain ingredients that can be toxic if ingested orally. When you make hand sanitizers at home and do not label them or keep them away from the kids, there is a chance of accidental ingestion that might prove hazardous. In case it does happen, it is advisable to take the child directly to the emergency room and inform them timely.

Illnesses like coronavirus or influenza have been seen to wreak havoc all across the world. An important thing to keep in mind is not to panic while the whole world is doing so. In this, we managed to educate you not only about the basics of hand sanitizer usage but also on the pros and cons and safety measures to take while using them. Remember, prevention is better than cure and together we can fight against any calamities that may befall.

W.H.O Recommended Hand Sanitizer Recipe

The WHO recommends that people use a hand sanitizer and give a recipe. This is the absolute best front-line protection for such diseases. These products appear to be an instrumental part of influenza control programs. They work on a variety of bacterial and viral diseases. Depending on what the agent is, it may be more, less tolerant, or prone to hand sanitizers.

However, for most things that people need to worry about in daily life (upper respiratory infections, gastrointestinal infections, and this type of thing), most of the factors that cause these diseases are highly vulnerable to modern hand sanitizers.

There are many, many hand sanitizer products on the market, but I have found that you can make your hand sanitizer at a fraction of the cost. Most of the products you buy are made from an alcoholic basis, but as green fashion continues, more natural products made from essential oils come to the market.

Essential oils have been used for thousands of years to combat the disease, and you may already have all the essential oils in your home to make hand sanitizer.

Tea tree oil is the most powerful of these antiseptics, but children or pregnant/lactating women should not use it. Adding more tea tree oil to any recipe will make hand sanitizer more effective, but the smell can be overwhelming.

In the recipes below, you can mix oils to suit your taste or just use one type of oil. Family safe aromatic oil blend option is a combination of lavender and pine. This will create a hand sanitizer with soothing effects.

Aloe vera gel is an ingredient in all of these recipes, and Ii is mention WHO that pure aloe vera gel without dyes or flavours. It is not like juice. It should be "100% aloe vera gel" in the bottle. If not, this is an error.

If you're having trouble finding any of these ingredients in your local stores, try the online resources. How to make your hand sanitizer with natural ingredients and what to buy when you don't want to make it yourself. This recipe produces approximately 2.5 ounces, which perfectly fit with these silicone bottles.

Preparation Time Is 5 Minutes

The ingredients

Pour the mixture(Aloe Vera gel cereal alcohol Vitamin E) into silicone bottles and place it in your wallet/purse for use on the go..

Notes

To use: Pour a small amount into the palm of your hand and knead with your hands, as needed. To turn this recipe into a hand sanitizer instead of gel, use five tablespoons of witch hazel extract instead of aloe vera and vodka/isopropyl alcohol. Ii is recommended using an alcohol-free version of this recipe.

If desired, add 1/2 teaspoon of vegetable glycerin to make the formula more hydrated. After adding the essential oils, pour it into a small spray bottle. Shake before use.

Handwashing Technique

Bloodborne pathogens can cause diseases in humans, and they are transmitted when infectious blood or other bodily fluid enters the body of another person. Exposure to bloodborne pathogens is more likely to occur in some work settings.

Infectious diseases are spread through unclean hands, so hand washing is prescribed as the most important practice to prevent or reduce the risk of infection and transmission.

Washing hands and other exposed skin as soon as possible after getting exposed to human blood, or other potentially infectious bodily fluids can help you get maximum protection.

Proper Hand Washing Techniques

Universal precautionary measures for preventing exposure to bloodborne pathogens insist that all human blood and bodily fluids should be treated as infectious, so it is crucial to take these measures immediately after contact with these substances.20

You can catch some infectious substances if you touch blood or other body fluids and touch your eyes, nose, or mouth without washing your hands properly.

Bloodborne pathogens may be transmitted through the mucous membranes of eyes, nose and mouth. Proper handwashing techniques can help prevent the risk of infection.

Use Soap And Water

It is important to use soap and water to wash your hands thoroughly, after treating wounds, giving medicine to a sick or injured person. You can use antibacterial soap and warm water to wash your hands.

Remove Jewelry Before Hand Washing

You should remove rings or any other jewellery pieces on the fingers and wrists, before washing your hands. Jewellery can interfere with sufficient cleansing.

Scrub Your Hands And Wrists

Wet your hands and wrists with warm water. Lather soap and scrub all the surfaces of your hands and wrists. Well. Scrubbing your hand with the palm of the other hand, can help remove all germs.

It is essential to rub in and between the fingers as well. Scrub the back of the hands thoroughly. Scrub each thumb and wrist by clasping in the opposite direction.

Spend 15-20 Seconds Washing Your Hands

Experts recommend spending 15 to 20 seconds washing your hands. Once you clean the hands perfectly, then rinse them with warm water.

Dry Your Hands

Pat your hands dry with a clean towel. You can also use a paper towel. Research studies say that wet hands can carry more infectious materials than dirty hands. A reusable cloth towel may have germs if it is not freshly laundered. If a clean cloth towel or new paper towel is not available, you can use air dryer to dry your hands.

Using Of Paper Towel To Turn Off The Faucet

The faucet may contain an infectious substance, so touching it after washing your hands can cause infection.

Small Things Matter

Make sure your sleeves are tight before you start washing your hands. They should not get wet during cleaning. Wash your forearms if you suspect they are contaminated.

In addition to proper handwashing, you should flush eyes, nose and mouth for 15 minutes, if blood or other bodily fluids are splashed in mucous membranes. These steps will help control the risk of infection as well as transmission.

Indoor sanitation: the exchange of air

The exchange of air inside the rooms of your home is important. It is necessary to: guarantee a good exchange of air in all environments: home or offices.

Not just private homes. By extending the discussion to closed places, even the themselves medical must provide for the exchange of air, as well as - especially in this period of high risk of infection ; the same pharmacies, banks, post, supermarkets and vehicles of transport.

To provide a correct exchange of air, it is sufficient to open the windows regularly, choosing those furthest from the busy streets. Instead, avoid opening them during peak traffic times and, above all, do not leave them open at night.

At the base of the sanitation activity is the activity of cleaning the rooms. When using cleaning products, follow the instructions indicated on each product, observing and respecting the dosages suggested on the packaging.

The various environments, materials and furnishings, in order to be well cleaned, can be treated with: water and soap and / or 75% ethyl alcohol and / or 0.5% sodium hypochlorite. In all cases, cleaning must be carried out with gloves or personal protective equipment.

It is important not to mix cleaning products, in particular those containing bleach or ammonia with other products and, both during and after the use of cleaning and sanitizing products, air the rooms.

Clean and disinfect surfaces

Among the most frequent questions regarding disinfection there is the one concerning denatured alcohol, that is the red type that since children has been recommended to us as a remedy to disinfect every small wound. This is because the alcohol that is usually found on the market, perhaps not at optimal concentrations, is mainly a bacteriostatic rather than a bactericide. This means that it serves to decrease the bacterial load by having a lighter antiseptic action. In any case, never apply it directly on organic matter because soap and water must first be used.

For example, if you want to consume the alcohol left in the house, before passing it on the kitchen surface, better wash it with water and soap or dishwashing detergent. Rinse and then also use alcohol.

There are also bleach or numerous other disinfectants for effective cleaning, but if the surface to be sanitized is not cleaned first, they have a reduced antibacterial capacity. So: it is always necessary to wash first, also in consideration of the fact that soap is a good antibacterial.

Capitolo 13 : Good Hygiene Practices

1. Hydrate, hydrate, hydrate! Be sure to drink plenty of water. Whether it be during your period, during exercise or lounging around. You can never go wrong with drink water. Spring water is the best option, it contains some minerals that can be absent in distilled and drinking water.

Your body is made up mostly of water, so it needs water to function properly. It hydrates the skin and most importantly, flushes out toxins and waste. It is the key to great health and hygiene.

Drink lots water should be a daily habit. The proper water intake is based on each individual. Take your weight and divide it in half. This magic number is the number of ounces you should be drinking daily:

For example, if I weigh 100 pounds, I would take that weight and divide that number in half which equals 50 pounds. I then use that number to find how many ounces of water I should drink daily. Remember this is the minimum you can always have more, especially if you exercise or are sweating a lot. Water is necessary, just think about it. Think of your body as a dishwasher full of dirty dishes. You won't have clean dishes if you don't have enough water.

2. Keep a separate laundry bag to place you dirty underwear and bras. If though you are washing your clothes you don't want your undergarments rubbing next to dirty street clothing. This is a great way for different bacteria and germs to be introduce to your private areas.

3. Wash you undergarments in skin sensitive washing detergent. Your privates are very delicate, sensitive areas and you will want to treat them as such. You not want to have harsh chemicals and perfumed soaps near those places. You have the option of using mild detergent, baby detergent or maybe use a lesser amount of detergent and rinse clothes twice.

4. Make sure underwear and bras are completely dry before wearing. The extra moisture is a breeding ground for bacteria to form which can cause things such as skin irritation, yeast infections and offensive odors.

5. Let your vagina breath. Take a break from wearing underwear and give it a chance to air out. Under wear traps that moisture in and can be somewhat suffocating. A perfect time to take a break is by sleeping commando (naked).

6. Going commando can be a very freeing feeling. However there are some instances when underwear is needed. Wearing undergarments under jeans is one of those instances. This is because jean can very tough and can be rough of your sensitive areas.

7. Cotton under wear is the best panty option. It is the most breathable, compared to its counterparts. Synthetic underwear like polyester can promote bad bacteria. Unfortunately, it seems the cutest underwear isn't usually the most hygienic, so wear them in moderation.

8. Wear thongs in moderation. Thongs floss their way into your crevices, making it harder for your private areas to ventilate properly.

9. The purpose of douching is to wash or clean out the vaginal canal. Douche cleanses are usually done after a menstrual cycle or sex. It is a common technique women use still, but doctors don't recommend it. Douching changes the delicate pH balance and cleanses away he healthy organisms in the vagina. Any changes can cause the overgrowth of bad bacteria leading to yeast infection and bacteria vaginosis. Also, if you are already infected, douching can push the infection in the ovaries and uterus.

10. Baby wipes are a great item to carry around in your pursue. They provide a cleaner feel than regular tissue. They can be used for multipurpose as well. They come in handy for makeup re-touches, a quick fleshing up and any small spills you may have. You can purchase feminine wipes but baby wipes work just as great but for half the price. The is also the option of flushable wipes, which makes for more convenience.

11. That time during your period can be very frustrating. Your mood swings, more that a pendulum and you just don't feel like our normal self. Keep your mind on other actives. Find a hobby or passion that you can put all of your attention towards. Engross yourself in a new project or learn a new skill. It can be something a bit challenging like learning a new language. On the other hand, it can be soothing and relaxing like

12. Alternating between hot and old showers can help stimulate blood circulation. The cold water causes the blood to rush to the organs to keep them warm. The hot warm causes the blood to rush to the skin so the vital organs do overheat. This process cleans out the lymph nodes and helps to remove toxins in the body that can cause bad odors.

    Start by showering in in warm to hot water, and shower regularly. Towards the end of the shower before you rinse the soap offer turn the water to cold. Maintain this temperature for 30 seconds and return to a comfortable temperature. Repeat this process a couple of more times. You will instantly feel energetic once you get out of the shower. The cold showers cause an energetic feel . Also if can opt to take only cold shower. The benefits of this are even better. Cols ware builds stringer immune system, hair follicles, clearer skin and better overall health.

13. You are what you eat. What you put inside reflects outward. It is simple concept but many people don't understand the significance that everything you do and do not put in your body will produce an effect. The food you eat effects your health, mood, appearance and your body scent. Eating clean gives you a clean and healthy scent. Keep in mind though that there are healthy foods such as onion and garlic that can produce an offense odor. However, most healthy foods allow the body to produce a natural aroma.

14. Greek yogurt can be used to cultivate good bacteria in your vagina. The vagina contains a host of organisms, which it uses to keep clean and healthy. This yogurt contains acidulous, which is a good bacteria. Make sure that it is PLAIN yogurt, because favored, sugar filled yogurt will only make the problem worse. Place the yogurt on a tampon and insert leave for 30 minutes then remove. Let the yogurt clean out by itself this should be done before bed as to avoid a mess of getting yogurt on your clothes.

15. Limit the amount of time spent in hot tubs and hot baths. Hot water can kill much of the natural bacteria in the vagina. The natural bacteria in the vagina is needed to maintain a healthy pH balance

16. Bubble bath is not vagina friendly. When sitting in a tub for extended period of time the dirt and soaps in the water can enter the vagina and cause pH imbalances. Use mild soaps. Try slicing

lemons and throwing those in your bath. Lemons provide a great smell, while not adversely affect the pH in the vagina.

17. If you use tampons be sure to replace them every few hours or when needed. A tampon is a foreign object and if let there to long can cause adverse effects. The body's immune system will try and attack the object and this can cause foul odors.

18. Frequently switching out your tampons will help make sure you don't develop toxic shock syndrome. This usually happens when a woman forgets to remove the tampon and the body reacts and cause her to be sick. This can be deadly.

19. Prepare a PMS emergency kit. Just in case of an emergency such as expected start of a period or other emergencies create a PMS kit. You can customize to your liking but here are some times that would be good include.

- 2 tampons in different sizes (regular, large, etc)
- 2 sanitary pads in different sizes (regular, super)
- baby wipes
- extra set of clean, dark underwear
- travel bottle baby powder
- favorite candy bar (comes in handy to calm for hankering cravings)
- aspirin

20. Remember to refill your kit and put it somewhere that you will have easy and immediate access to. You can place the items in a small durable bag and put it in the truck of your car, desk in your office, somewhere conveniently discreet.

21. Lowering you sugar intake not only helps keep the pounds off but also help with vaginal help. Too much sugar can can overproduction of yeast in the vagina. Bacteria feeds on sugar and too much of the bacteria can cause imbalances. You can also combat these by upping your water intake.

22. Wipe front to back, front to back, FRONT to BACK! Use this motion to wipe yourself clean when using the restroom. This will prevent any bacteria from your anal region to infiltrate your vagina.

23. Removing or trimming hair can help in hygiene. Places where there is a lot of hair and moisture can be a harvesting ground for odors to develop. Places like your private area and underarms and other crevices like these can sweat and produce moisture easily. This places also have a lot of hair. The sweat and odors attach to the hair causing odor to linger.

24. Shower loofahs are a good washing tool to use in the shower. They help to loosen the dirt and exfoliate the skin. They also aid in lathering soap, which will help your soap to last longer.

25. Make your perfume last longer by layering. Of course you will need to start with a fresh palette and cleanse the skin. While in the shower use a scented shampoo and body wash or soap. Lather the soap on the body from head to toe, very well. Step from under the shower head for 30 seconds or longer and allow the scent to sink into the skin. Rinse the body and then precede toward step two. After you are out of the shower and dried off, take a body spray and mist the body form head to toe. A few light spritz here, a few spritz there, nothing major. Next, apply a scented lotion over the body. After this spritz perfume, which as a heavier longer lasting scent, as the final step.

26. A nice bottle of perfume can be costly. Using your perfume efficiently will ensure that you get the most from your perfume. Applying the perfume to "hot spots", on the body will allow the perfume to last longer and smell stronger. This "hot spots" are called pulse points. These are areas on the body that are especilly warm. The back of the neck, behind the knee, infornt of the elbow

27. Feminine wash is only eat to clean the exterior of the vagina. Using these kinds of products inside the vagina can cause pH imbalances and irritation.

28. Of course, you already know to brush your teeth morning and night. But if you are able, brush your teeth after every meals and especially after desserts.

29. Be sure to floss often and gargle with antiseptic mouthwash. Tilt your head back and swish the mouthwash for a minimum of 60 seconds or sing the alphabet song, so it can have time to clean properly.

30. Sometimes during a menstrual cycle, there can be accidents and spills. As soon as possible before putting in the washer soak the article of clothing.

31. Blood stains can be easily removed by soaking the article of clothing is cold water. If any stains remain, add a ½ teaspoon dish-washing or liquid laundry detergent and a tablespoon of monomial for 15 minutes.

33. Schedule a wash day. This is a day dedicated to washing your clothes. Keeping a schedule will insure you will always have clean clothes and will help you to not get overwhelmed if you let clothes pile up.

34. Sort your whites, pastels and lights into a pile separate from dark.

- Use Regular/Normal wash cycle

- Hot water scalds the stains from the white clothing

- Bleach is used to get tough stains out

- Baking soda and borax

    35. It is best when sorting colors to put like colors together, if possible

- pink, reds, oranges, yellows

- yellows, greens, blues

- greens, blues, purples

- purples, browns, blacks

- Use cold water to help preserve the vibrancy of the color.

    35. White baths towels and face cloths are recommended as they contain no color dyes that colored clothes have. This is important as it limits the amount of chemicals that you are using to clean your body. Also, white towels are easier to clean because you can bleach them. Some towels even after being washed can contain mildew and dirt residue. Using such a strong cleaner ensures that you get them as clean as possible.

    36. Most people after purchasing new clothes precede to bring them straight from the store to their clothes. It is important to remember just because they are purchased from the store doesn't mean they haven't been worn before. The article of clothing may have been tried on by other customers. This is especially true for pants and bottoms. You don't want to expose your body to stranger's fluids and dirt. Be sure to wash and disinfect your new clothes, before wearing, just to be on the safe side.

37. Exfoliation is the process of removing the oldest dead skin cells on the skin's outermost surface. This technique is used f to help maintain healthy, polished skin. There are numerous ways to buffer the skin and can create a cleaner, hygienic skin. Exfoliation buffers away the barrier of dead skin cells that clogs the pores. So removing the dead cells allows lotions and oils to better absorb into the skin.

38. Dry body brushing is one of the best and cheapest ways to exfoliate the skin. You can find a body brush at most places where you purchases other beauty supplies. You can brush on a daily basis, preferably right before showering. Began by brushing the feet in circular motions and work your way upward toward the heart. Dry brushing promotes circulation through out the body. The brushing exfoliates by sloughing off dead skin cells and revealing a new, radiant layer of skin.

39. Coffee grinds are another way to remove dead skin. Combine two cups of coffee grinds with enough honey until the moisture is a think liquid consistency. Wet skin the in the shower and apply the concoction in circular motions. This not only leaves skin soft but helps to combat cellulite. The caffeine stimulates the fat cells in the thighs and but which helps to reduce cellulite. So concentrate rubbing these areas for best results. Rinse and continue with your normal shower routine.

40. Exercising is great for overall health. It creates endorphins, a good feeling hormone, and creates a more desirable physique. Exercising also helps to release toxins through sweating, which ultimately leaving the body more hygienic..

41. White teeth are not only are more attractive but are a sign of good heath and hygiene. There a different methods cheap and costly to brighten teeth. You gave the option of going to a dentist and getting them whitened. This process can cost upwards to hundreds of dollars. You can by whitening trips and trays. Or you can use more holistic and inexpensive, yet effect ways to achieve a brighter smile.

    Combine hydrogen peroxide and baking soda to create a paste. Dip tooth brush in the solution and brush teeth as you would normally. Repeat the process several times a week for whiter teeth.

    Instead of buying a tooth whitening tray you can make your own. Purchase a plastic mouth guard like the ones athletes use, from your local store. Bring some water to a boil and place the mouth guards into the water for a few seconds until hey are soft and pliable. Once they are gummy-like place into mouth over teeth. Begin to form the guard around your teeth. Bite down and suck the air from out of the guard. Once removed from the mouth, you should be left with a mold of your teeth. This personalized mouth tray can be filled with teeth whiting gel.

Another method of lightning teeth is by creating a mixture of lemon juice and salt until it forms a paste. Apply to the teeth alike toothpaste. The abrasive salt will remove plaque from teeth while the lemon provides deep cleansing.

42. Sanitary napkins are worn during a woman's period to collect the blood her body expels. This fluid over time can create an offense odor, and therefore should be replaced often. These pads should be changed every two to three hours depending on the heaviness of the menstrual flow.
43. Baby powder can be used as a deodorant to combat odors. It also helps to cut down on bacteria formation by absorbing the moisture that are located in damp crevices of the body.
44. Eating a plum right before bed helps in preventing morning breath.
45. Always keep a pack of gum, or Listerine strips on hand, to pop in your mouth for a quick breathe freshener.
46. If you are in public and need to brush your teeth and do not have a tooth brush opt for the portable tooth brushes. Colgate makes on the-go tooth brushes.
47. Treat any oral diseases. Cavities and oral diseases can cause bad breath. They also can lead to heart disease and other health problems.
48. Keep a pumice stone in near the shower and run it across the soles of your feet to prevent dry and rough feet. The pumice will buffer the rough texture on the soles of the fee

to reveal soft smooth skin. Add a dot of liquid soap and scrub for 1-2 minutes.

Capitolo 14 : Conclusion

When it comes to making home- made hand sanitizers in order to fight germs and stay healthy, it is important to get it right so as to enjoy its maximum benefits.

With the whole panic about the outbreak of infectious diseases in the last decade, it has become imperative that we all kick our hygiene levels up a notch and stay healthy.

Thanks to numerous efforts by experts and the guidance of reputable health organizations, following various recipes can help you formulate skin- friendly, effective hand sanitizers. This can help you significantly cut down on your budget when it comes to purchasing branded hand-sanitizing products which have become increasingly scarce and outrightly expensive.

As much as these recipes can be highly effective, the following points ought to be noted:

- Washing of hands with soap remains the best singular action for maintaining absolute cleanliness. The use of hand sanitizers should be restricted to only when soap and water are not available. This act of washing hands with soap must

- be done regularly and properly- ever so often and lasting for up to a minimum of 20 seconds.
- It is important to continuously check with registered medical personnel or healthcare provider before using essential oils, particularly when it comes to children or in the case where you are nursing a medical condition.
- Fresh aloe vera gel isn't very stable when it comes to storage; so, it is recommended that you explore commercial brands of aloe vera in the market.
- Some alcohol concentrates can be harmful when ingested or when it comes in contact with the eyes. If it gets into the eyes, it is recommended that you flush eyes with plenty of water and seek immediate medical attention. Use gloves when handling such concentrates.
- These recipes are not in any way to be taken as standard prescriptions or anything close to that. They are subject to further evaluations and must be used with discretion.
- The concentration of alcohol within your recipes is to be followed strictly. Do not go below WHO recommendations as these may render your final products ineffective.
- Alcohol- free hand sanitizers have been shown to be effective but can cause some germs to become intolerant. So, it is recommended that your recipes do contain alcohol as recommended by WHO

- Keep your home-made hand sanitizers, as well as other medical product away from the reach of children. do consult a doctor immediately in the event that a child accidentally ingests the product

In fact, There are countless recipes for hand sanitizers. The idea, though, should be that any recipes should remain within the boundaries of standard medical recommendations and efficiency.

It is important that you do not trade appearance for quality or pleasant aromas for efficiency. Also, do not experiment with ingredients without precautionary measure put in place. This might end up badly, and you could get hurt. Always remember that the main objective of attempting to put up any product in the first place is to keep you safe.

So, as you experiment, be curious, resolute, yet careful, precise and flawless. Be safe.

We are being frightened by graphic marketing from the manufacturers of these items to eliminate all bacteria or somewhat 99.9% lest we fall for the target to colds, flu, or any type of viral illness. We are motivated to 'safeguard' our family members against the marauding, unseen bacteria.

I would certainly like you to take into consideration how the overuse of anti-bacterial products from hand sanitizers to emerge sprays as well as cleansers, might, over time, impact our immune system as well as for that reason essential wellness. A number of the active ingredients in the items have not been thoroughly checked for human safety, while others, via research, reveal poisoning even at reduced doses.

Surprisingly, a research study by the University of Virginia has shown that alcohol-based hand sanitizers didn't considerably decrease the variety of individuals contaminated with a cold or flu. Of 100 volunteers that used a hand sanitizer, 54 ended up being unwell with a cool or flu, while 66 of 100 people that did not utilize it experienced a virus.

What is shocking is that while lots of people believe hand sanitizers are active and also effective for a very long time after application, alcohol sanitizers last just a min or two and also must be reapplied when recontamination takes place.

Even the U.S. Center for Condition Control confesses that hand sanitizers will not kill all bacteria. As well as when reading the ingredients tag of a hand sanitizer, the listing consists of several active ingredients, not yet evaluated for safety and security in cosmetics. The remainder has actually been found to be toxic irritants, health hazards, and contaminants.

Include in that information is a study from scientists from the National College of Ireland that discovered a typical disinfectant and also antimicrobial representative made use of in hand sanitizers, benzalkonium chloride has actually revealed the capacity to establish a resistance to some antibiotics. The researchers located that by adding increasing amounts of the disinfectant to germs, not just do the bacteria survive the chemical, however additionally a generally used antibiotic, ciprofloxacin, even when the checked germs have actually not been exposed to the antibiotic.

And also, there is even more problematic for benzalkonium chloride, as the chemical is believed human immune system toxicant, breathing system irritant, have reproduction & development results, eye and also a skin irritant and also can create stomach distress if consumed. So simply do not make use of a product with this chemical as an ingredient if you intend to handle food or water, or touch your eyes or lips.

The chemical is yet to be figured out safe for pregnant and also nursing women or youngsters under the age of 2. Benzalkonium chloride is the main reason for bronchial asthma and also dermatitis in health care workers as well as specialist cleaning personnel.

Triclosan is an additional preferred ingredient in sanitizers, both individual and home products. This chemical is hazardous to humans, impacting the thyroid and also various other hormonal agent systems. A study on a cross-section of the American population detected triclosan in the pee of 75% of the greater than 2500 people checked. In another research carried out by the Mount Sinai Institution of Medicine, the chemical was detected in the pee of 61% of 90 ladies matured from 6 to 8 years.

Triclosan infects the water as well as the atmosphere ways it is flushed into from wastewater therapy plants as it cannot be entirely eliminated. It is harmful to wild animals and also aquatic pets from algae to fish. Researchers have discovered traces of triclosan in 58% of 85 streams in the UNITED STATES.

Triclosan engages with sunshine as well as microorganisms in surface water to develop methyl triclosan, a chemical that may bio accumulate in wildlife and also human beings.

Alcohol, either ethyl or isopropyl, is the major as well as an active ingredient in hand sanitizers, composing more than 60% of the whole product. It is the alcohol that eliminates the bacteria and also infections.

Nevertheless, ethyl alcohol is an infiltration booster, taking the other chemicals deeper into the skin as well as into the bloodstream. Not ideal if the other ingredients are toxic and even doubtful.

Isopropyl alcohol, likewise called scrubbing alcohol, is from the petrochemical sector, is extremely drying out, and also is harmful to the nerves. It is absorbed via the skin and also from the breathing of the vapors.

The scent is made use of in everything. We are also motivated to buy instruments that will provide consistent puffs of fabricated fragrance right into our house to make them scent 'fresh'! But these fragrances can be comprised of greater than 4000 various chemicals, most of them poisonous. It is recognized that these chemicals can collect in the body. Phthalates, utilized to make certain the scent lingers longer, are recognized hormone disruptors. Scientists have actually researched the results of phthalates on baby kids as well as have proof that they disturb the babies' sexual advancement.

These are just a few of the ingredients in hand sanitizers; you might be tired if I detailed as well as clarify them all. So, are we actually incoming a war versus bacteria? Or are we being suckered into yet another item to add to the shopping list, fearful that we may be on the brink of a health and wellness taking the chance of an epidemic?

It has actually been shown by countless wellness research studies that great old soap, as well as water, is more effective in cleansing hands than packaged hand sanitizers, without the possible threats of adding yet much more chemicals to our bodies and also right into the atmosphere.

Add to that the positive effect on the immune system in building anti-bodies to naturally fight disease and I'd say we can well do without these little bottles of poison that are rapidly multiplying throughout the world.

Remember, even according to the manufactures, hand sanitizers only kill 99.9% of germs… what happens to the remaining .1%?

They mutate and become stronger, eventually resisting all methods of killing them.

Myths and Misconceptions about hand sanitizers.

There are various misconceptions and myths regarding hand sanitizers. Within this guide, we are going to have a look at a few details to debunk the myths and put the record right.

Among the most well-known misconceptions is that hand sanitizers are almost infallible, and they can stop the spread of contagious diseases, for instance, cold or influenza. Even though a hand sanitizer may kill over 60% of influenza viruses onto your hands, many people really contract influenza from airborne representatives, by breathing at the germs. Thus, even in the event that you've employed a sterile merchandise, and your hands are fresh and germ-free, you're still able to catch or spread the virus. A hand sanitizer might actually be much stronger preventative mechanism for gastrointestinal ailments, instead of illnesses like the flu or cold.

The other myth is they are much less effective as traditional handwashing with soap and water, also in eliminating germs in your hands on. This isn't always correct. Washing with water and soap functions betters in case your hands are obviously soiled, in other words, in case you've got dirt from your hands. But in case your hands look fresh but are now intercepted using germs; subsequently, an alcohol-based hand sanitizer is still a better choice since the alcohol is significantly more successful in eliminating the germs.

The next myth is that hand sanitizers cause dry hands. These products include emollients that are compounds that reduce aggravation by soothing and protecting skin. As counterintuitive as it might look, an alcohol-based hand sanitizer is really less harsh on skin than soap and water. A research conducted by Brown University researchers found that washing your hands with water and soap contributes to skin, which may appear and feel very dry. A hand sanitizer on the opposite hand can keep hands sterile.

You're able to earn a somewhat powerful sanitizer in the home. While homemade versions might be more economical, most do not include the recommended 60 percent alcohol content, which experts agree is that the best concentration to get rid of germs. The best results are observed with new names, for example, Purell or even Germ X.

However, provided that the item includes 60% alcohol, some generic manufacturer may work just as good as a superior store brand new. You do not need to pay the high cost for a brand name merchandise.

Compiling all of the hand sanitizer truth, we may safely state an alcohol-based sanitizer has become easily the best ways to kill germs from our own hands but just provided that the item is used properly and efficiently.

Alcohol-based sanitizer isn't just able to remove more germs than water and soap, but it's also gentler in skin when used in moderate quantities. When supervised by an adult, this item could be safe for children too.

While alcohol-based sanitizers have confronted criticism of late, but largely as a result of alcohol concentration, specialists say that a few of those fears are unfounded. Alcohol isn't absorbed into skin into some level to justify these anxieties. In spite of excessive utilization, the degree of alcohol consumption is benign in the top. Alcohol can contribute to a sanitizer risks, but not to any wonderful extent.

The debate against alcohol material only holds up when the goods are employed in a manner, they weren't meant to be utilized in. By way of instance, an alcohol-based hand sanitizer isn't supposed to be consumed; however, there have been a number of instances where children in addition to adults have swallowed the liquid and dropped very sick.

Some producers have tried to deal with the public's concern over alcohol material and began producing alcohol-free versions as a safer choice. These products rely upon plant oils neutralize germs, but to date haven't been as successful as alcohol-based hand sanitizers. If utilized correctly, an alcohol-based hand sanitizer isn't any more harmful than an alcoholic free version.

To protect yourself against viruses and bacteria, the best defense remains prevention.

Compliance with basic hygiene rules and minor health precautions can help you prevent or avoid infection.

Bringing your hands to your face or mouth is a habitual, often involuntary gesture, but you should avoid it because it facilitates the transmission and entry of pathogens into your body.

Nose, eyes and mouth are in fact the main gateway for viruses and bacteria.

In the fight against the spread of infectious diseases, washing your hands frequently and carefully is one of the most recommended, simple and effective prevention measures.

Viruses, bacteria, mites, pollen and all pathogens that threaten your health can also be found in large quantities inside the home and in private transport, such as cars and motorhomes, which you use daily. To clean and remove dirt you are used to using chemical sprays and detergents, but for deeper cleaning and to eliminate germs and allergens, there is no better way to sanitize the environment than with homemade disinfectants using natural, non-chemical ingredients.

www.ingramcontent.com/pod-product-compliance
Lightning Source LLC
Chambersburg PA
CBHW071402210526
45465CB00001B/211